Canadian Medicare

+

Canadian Medicare

We Need It and We Can Keep It

+

Stephen Duckett and Adrian Peetoom

McGill-Queen's University Press

Montreal & Kingston · London · Ithaca

Legal deposit first quarter 2013
Bibliothèque nationale du Québec

Printed in Canada on acid-free paper that is 100% ancient forest free
(100% post-consumer recycled), processed chlorine free

McGill-Queen's University Press acknowledges the support of the Canada
Council for the Arts for our publishing program. We also acknowledge the
financial support of the Government of Canada through the Canada Book
Fund for our publishing activities.

The authors wish to thank the School of Policy at Queen's University
for its support of this book.

Library and Archives Canada Cataloguing in Publication

Duckett, S. J.
Canadian medicare : we need it and we can keep it / Stephen
Duckett and Adrian Peetoom.

Includes bibliographical references and index.
ISBN 978-0-7735-4154-2

1. National health insurance – Canada. 2. Health care reform – Canada.
I. Peetoom, Adrian II. Title.

RA412.5.C3D83 2013   362.10971   C2012-907565-5

This book was designed and typeset by studio oneonone in Sabon 11/14

Contents

Canadian Medicare

A Call to Action

There is no shortage of proposals for health care reform. Most take the general approach you will find in this book. Recommendations similar to many of ours may be found in older books, in newspaper and journal articles, in letters to the editor, and in conference speeches and have been raised in informal conversations among health care professionals. Here is a clear recent example, found in the *Globe and Mail* on April 17, 2012, on page A3 in an article by André Picard: "We need to fix our fundamental approach to delivering care – to put the emphasis on managing chronic disease and caring for people in the community and take it away from the outmoded approach to providing all acute care in institutions."

This book makes this point and others as well. We also consider the following question: Even though here and there positive changes are being made, why have a whole series of well-known and well-researched improvements in medicare not been widely implemented in all Canadian provinces and territories? We have a simple but complex answer. Canadians have not yet put enough pressure on politicians and health care professionals. If citizens are to exert such pressure, they need to be aware of the bundle of major new directions required to sustain and improve medicare initiatives. That is why we wrote this book for all Canadians. It provides material for an informed public discussion. It is also an invitation to ordinary citizens to get more involved in preserving and improving this part of our national identity. All of us have a substantial stake in maintaining a well-functioning and sustainable Canadian medicare system that will improve our health and help us cope better with the frailties of aging. Moreover, if more Canadians know what is possible within the current value system of a publicly funded universal health system, then ideas that undermine and threaten that system will get less traction.

But we also ask: If it is already widely known how medicare may be sustained and improved, why is there so much talk of a crisis? Why are many Canadians worried about the future of medicare? Why do waiting times not seem to shrink? Why are middle and lower income seniors worried about what will happen to them when they need some degree of permanent care?

These and other anxious questions that are regularly being asked in the letters to the editor pages of our major newspapers keep coming up because knowing what needs to happen is one thing, but making it happen is another. As Picard observed in the same article, "Sadly, [the important questions] don't get discussed because we are too busy tilting quixotically at windmills like privatization instead of slaying the real dragons in the health-care system." This book seeks to change the agenda. Health care professionals are responsible for making the necessary changes – "making it happen." But they will act boldly only when politicians get pushed and prodded by ordinary Canadians. This book provides non-professionals with the knowledge they will need to play their own crucial role in preserving and improving medicare. Each chapter is a call to action. Politicians need to enable health care professionals to implement new ways of providing care, ways that are well researched and documented. They will act only when we ordinary Canadians urge them to do so.

Our medicare is an important piece in the puzzle of Canadian life. It is an emphatically positive answer to the question, "Am

I my Canadian brother's/sister's keeper?" Medicare is NOT largess from a generous government (although politicians are forever pretending it is). It is also NOT an insurance policy (even though the word insurance is part of the *Canada Health Act*). Both Tommy Douglas and Lester Pearson, builders of Canadian medicare and politicians with insight and courage, believed that medicare was a way for all Canadians to share burdens when illness threatens to overwhelm personal and family finances. Medicare is a simple idea, really. We all contribute a reasonable amount of money to a fund, out of which we pay doctors and other health care professionals to help us maintain and improve our health and restore it when threatened. That's the gist of it.

The authors of this book bring different experiences to this project. Stephen Duckett, an Australian whose wife is Canadian, brings a professional life spent examining the complex systems that sustain the simple idea of medicare. He is an internationally respected Australian economist who has made investigating the workings of medicare his life's work. He has worked in the public sector all his professional life, in hospitals, universities, government, and health authorities. He is in constant demand as a university lecturer and consultant advising governments and health care institutions. For a time he was president and CEO of Alberta Health Services, the umbrella organization in charge of Alberta's health care system. Unfortunately his time for implementing necessary changes was cut short, but his research and Canadian experience are summarized in his recently published book entitled *Where to from Here? Keeping Medicare Sustainable* (Montreal and Kingston: Queen's Policy Studies and McGill-Queen's University Press, 2012).

Adrian Peetoom brings specific memories of his early immigrant days in Canada. As an eager nineteen-year-old he came to our beautiful land in March 1954. Within a month, and without advance warning, he had to have his appendix removed. He was faced with the following financial consequences, which overwhelmed the $15 in his pocket, all he had:

1   The family doctor of his landlord got him to a hospital in his own car. His normal fee for care, that day and afterward, was $50, but knowing Adrian's circumstances, the doctor waived it.
2   The surgeon's fee was $150, but he cut it in half at the request of the family doctor. Adrian paid the $75 bit by bit, often with the proceeds of odd jobs on Saturdays with wages of about $1 per hour.
3   The anesthesiologist waved his fee, also at the urging of the family doctor.
4   The hospital charged $260 and didn't back down for as much as a penny. For six months Adrian walked to the hospital every Saturday morning and left $10 lighter, until the bill was paid.

What's the big deal? Doesn't seem that big of a burden, does it? But consider the math. Adrian worked at a bank for the princely sum of $26 per week. Of this, $15 went to his landlord for room and board. With $10 going to the hospital, there was $1 left per week for all other expenses. Adrian didn't have enough money for bus fare, so he walked 40 minutes to and from work each day. He didn't have any money for outings, movies, concerts, or recreation that required money, not even a quarter for an occasional coffee and slice of his favourite lemon meringue pie at a cafe. Fortunately his immigrant church stepped in and contributed what it could out of its own meager resources to buy him clothes more suitable to a harsh Canadian winter.

Adrian was single and basically healthy. This surgical mishap may have robbed him of some financial freedom for a while, but it didn't kill his plans for the future. However, he saw other immigrant families having to face far worse health problems, with more devastating financial consequences. One or two lost a child, some fathers couldn't earn a living because of illness or a serious accident but they still had to cope with a stack of medical bills, and some mothers were unable to look after their (often quite large) families. For all of those families the prospect of a national medicare program, realized in the early 1960s, was a huge relief.

Stephen has his own memories of scrambling for money to pay for care. His sister had a serious illness when she was young and his family had to sell the land on which it had hoped to build the first family home to pay for her care. He was hospitalized a few years later, further setting back the family finances.

Rare is the extended family that hasn't been hit with illness, either acute or chronic. Although Canadians have been fortunate in experiencing the benefits of medicare, many of us have seen the devastation (bankruptcy and family disintegration) that serious illness can bring to our American relatives and friends. And we are troubled, if not bewildered, by the frequent reports that Canadian medicare is in trouble. Some say that as a nation we may not be able to sustain it. We hear two-tiered care being proposed as an option, about the Americanization of our health care system, about people of wealth and influence being able to jump the queue (e.g., professional athletes getting MRIs the day of an injury). Many Canadians are already financially pressed and fear that the critics may be right: the day will come when medicare will shrink, and illness will once more have serious financial consequences.

Health care touches everyone. The health care sector attracts people who want to make a difference in the lives of individuals, communities, and society as a whole. Some make a health care profession their life's work. Some give of their time and energy as volunteers, providing comfort or advice. People with a chronic illness use health care a lot, and their friends and families are often intimately involved as well. All of us derive comfort from the thought that care will be available when we require it, and because we're all part of medicare, it attracts lots of scrutiny. Given that medicare is the business of all Canadians, we all need to have some insight into the policy issues that affect it so that we can better equip ourselves to push and prod politicians to invest in best practices for health care professionals to sustain and improve our medicare and to focus on real challenges, not on imagined ones, even though the latter ones may be politically and professionally profitable.

This book is a defense of medicare and a call to arms to improve it. The two elements go hand in hand: without improvements, it will become much more difficult to sustain medicare. We will address the following kinds of questions over and over again, in various contexts.

- What's going on in medicare, and how does its current form differ from medicare years ago?
- What are critics of medicare saying, and how should we respond to them?
- What are the most important challenges to medicare, both in terms of maintaining it and improving it?
- What (and who) needs to change?

As you read this book, you will encounter several motifs that express ideas to which we are committed.

- We think that all Canadians have a stake in the health of all other Canadians. The heart of medicare is a resounding "yes" to the question, "Am I my brother's/sister's keeper?"
- For medicare to be maintained and improved, the commitment and competence of health care providers (physicians, nurses, other professionals,

administrators, support staff) are crucial. All of them must be given room to become the best they can at their jobs.
- Every Canadian has responsibility to safeguard his or her own health.
- Politicians have but one function with respect to health care: to enable professionals to do their work with the greatest possible social efficiency. Social efficiency has to do with achieving the most positive outcomes at an affordable cost. Social efficiency in health care means Canadians living longer and healthier lives with a minimum of suffering.

We particularly want to stress the second motif. Neither of us is involved in the day-to-day intricacies of providing health care to those in need – only health care professionals are. And so this book is also a call to arms to those professionals: we call on them to roll up their sleeves, put their shoulders to the wheel, and do whatever it takes to preserve and improve medicare. This book not only says that they should but that they can and that they will enjoy working at improving medicare as a better expression of their education, training, and complex skills. While desires for career success, compensation, and respect play roles in their decision making, their commitment is a commitment of the heart, a desire to relive the stress of people in distress.

The Point of this Book

We want to help ordinary Canadians become more familiar with the ins and outs of the medicare we all share. We're not asking them to fix and improve it; professionals and politicians take the lead on that. Our hope is that ordinary Canadians will be a bit more savvy about medicare after reading this book and will be able to put pressure on those politicians and professionals to sustain and improve medicare. Improvements are needed not just in terms of costs, taxes, and the range of services covered, but also, importantly, in terms of enabling medicare to help us all have a longer, healthier life.

In 2014, the ten-year health accord signed in 2004 that governed the annual flow of medicare money from the federal government to the provinces and territories will come to an end. The federal government has already announced the next financial settlement. Federal coffers will provide two more years of 6% increases in health transfer payments, but after that increases will be tied to the gross domestic product (GDP). Federal officials have said there will be no strings attached, and each province or territory can use the funds in the ways it sees fit. This means that ordinary Canadians need to focus on what their provinces have in mind.

In each province and territory, pundits point to the fact that health care costs have been rising faster than increases in the GDP for several years, thereby commanding ever increasing portions of total provincial budgets. Questions are being asked: Is that trend unstoppable? Is medicare sustainable? Changes are necessary, but can they be made within the framework of the existing principles of medicare, or should we revisit, and perhaps redraft, those principles? What about two-tiered health care? Is our medicare a voracious and out-of-control monster devouring public budgets and demanding ever increasing tax revenues? What about our aging population and the threats posed by conditions such as obesity? These and other questions are tackled in this book. Rest assured that the responses are firmly grounded in research. Every claim made in this book can be substantiated.

Before anyone gets overly anxious, we want to share this bit of encouraging news. Survey after survey shows that the vast majority of Canadians support health care that is universally and equitably accessible and publicly financed. Almost every let-

ter to the editor discussing a problem encountered by the let-
ter writer, perhaps concerning waiting times and the shortage of
family doctors, is followed by one or more letters in which the
writer lauds the system on the basis of personal experiences.
Most of these submissions take the form of personal stories,
either positive or negative: health is always a very personal matter, ultimately. That is why former Saskatchewan premier Roy
Romanow called medicare "a defining aspect of our citizenship." Medicare is ours, and we're willing to take care of it.
Politicians and health care professionals have central caring
roles, and most of them understand that they must use their
knowledge and skill to serve us all. Still, all politicians need to
know that we ordinary Canadians consider medicare ours: we
want it and we need it. Of course, as we shall also argue, we
all need to realize that we are responsible for doing all we can
to avoid being an unnecessary drain on the system.

The question of sustainability is a legitimate one and should
be part of both the political agenda and our personal reflections.
This book argues that our medicare is sustainable. What do
we mean by sustainable? Simply this: our economy can bear the
cost of it, now and in the future, without the need to impose
extraordinary taxes and without jeopardizing other essential
services like education. Moreover, medicare, as we see it, will be
able to provide Canadians with the care they need, even when
the projected increase in chronic conditions has its impact, and
with new technologies (pharmaceuticals and procedures) being
developed all the time. There is no need for substantial private
funding. There is no need to change the five criteria that govern provincial medicare arrangements (see chapter 1). There is
no need to ask Canadians to weaken their commitment to medicare. There is no need to sacrifice access, quality, or sustainability; all three elements can be maintained. However, we need
to harness uncontrolled spending and to be prudent investors of
our health care dollars. We need to manage better and to provide

services efficiently and without waste. The future of medicare is about making wise investments in health care. Without wise investments medicare's fundamentals will be undermined, so this work must be done.

As you read this book you will come to realize that we are not laying down a precise prescription for a new medicare, which, if followed (or "swallowed") will make all problems disappear. Instead, we diagnose problem areas and then invite politicians and professionals to go to work. We are convinced that addressing most human problems requires the combined and cooperative efforts of those who are on the front lines. We believe in teamwork, and we have confidence in the skills of professionals. Ordinary Canadians need to know more about positive options that will ensure a universal public system that is based on values we share. Medicare is sustainable, and in this book we provide the information Canadians need to hold the professionals and politicians to account.

Here is how the book is organized.

- In chapter 1 we review the legislative underpinnings of our health care system: the *Canada Health Act*, the 2004 health accord, and current provincial health care funding systems.
- In chapter 2 we meet the sustainability doubts head on. We make the case that we need not give in to economic doubts. We deal with Canada's demographic trends and the impact of an aging population on health care costs.
- In chapter 3 we discuss the problems of financial sustainability and suggest ways of responding to them.
- In chapters 4–9 we carefully review a number of major health care initiatives meant to improve patient care and the financial stability of the system. Key is the switch from a traditional acute care

approach to a more relevant chronic care approach. Health care has undergone a fundamental change in the last fifty years, from focusing on acute care to focusing on chronic care, but health care structures have barely begun to respond to that change. We need to take a good look at the use of primary care, varied programs for seniors, the function and place of hospitals, and the use of pharmaceuticals and other technologies. For each of these areas, wise investments will produce substantial long-term savings. We need to expand primary care clinics for everyone and provide assisted living facilities for seniors.

- In chapter 10 we address planning for appropriate staffing. We argue that we need a much more varied health care workforce.
- In chapter 11 we provide a forum for critics and stakeholders, and we provide our reactions to their views.
- In chapter 12 we summarize what we have learned and point the way to a solid future for medicare.

To keep this book as readable as possible, references, charts, and tables are kept to a minimum, and we provide acknowledgments of sources only when we directly cite other authors. The term "provinces" encompasses both provinces and territories unless otherwise specified.

CHAPTER 1

Our Medicare Structure in Broad Strokes

Medicare is more than laws and regulations. As the Romanow report (2002) pointed out, from the beginning medicare has been an expression of our care for one another. As some other writers have said, it is as binding an element of Canadian life today as the railroads that connected East and West in the nineteenth century. Our medicare is a commitment Canadians made to one another more than half a century ago. In times of need brought on by health problems, we will continue to help each other financially. Medicare is ours. It is not the beneficence of governments, be they federal or provincial. Nor is it the goodwill of health care corporations. However much appreciated, it is not even the kindness of front-line health care professionals: physicians, nurses, equipment technicians, medical administrators, and hospital orderlies. All those simply represent the will of the people fed by a spirit of generosity and care for one another.

Canadians sometimes forget this fact, and who can blame them? In a country as large as ours, with a population steadily growing and now well over 33 million, we need complex organization to give expression to our generosity. Our generosity gets to be mediated, almost overshadowed, by organizations. Many hospitals and drug companies are involved, and these institutions often obey their own primary rule: "got to be looking good." Governments want to appear to be the source of citizen wellness, be it economic, social, or medical. Drug companies stress the presumed benefits of their chemicals and suppress their often highly questionable marketing strategies. Physicians don't always possess superb bedside manners, and some believe they hold the key to unlocking the secrets of the human body and must be regarded with a special type of awe. However, the work of all of these contributors to the health care system, even the kindest of nurses, only happens because of the generosity of the more than 33 million neighbours who share our country, those we know and those we don't know: our tax dollars pay for all of the costs of the Canadian health care system. This generosity sets the context for our medicare and must be kept in mind in any discussion about how to change the system.

That context is expressed in three major institutional ways:

- The *Canada Health Act* defines our medicare.
- The 2004 health accord provided a ten-year regulated flow of funds (our taxes) from Ottawa to provincial governments and described the agreed level of services.
- For the daily operation of medicare, provincial governments provide a steady stream of regulations about the funding of professionals and set guidelines for them.

Let's look at all three in more detail.

The *Canada Health Act* (1984)

In our federal system of government, the federal government has a limited role in health care. Our constitution gives the provinces exclusive power over hospitals. Each province's jurisdiction is contained within its own provincial borders. Only with respect to health as a national issue can Ottawa make laws. Hence the

Canada Health Act sets out health care provisions that apply to all Canadians. However, the provinces are responsible for the details of the act's implementation. Here is how the *Canada Health Act* articulates the broad "primary objective of Canadian health care policy": "to protect, promote and restore the physical and mental well-being of residents of Canada and to facilitate *reasonable access* to health services without financial or other barriers" (section 3, emphasis added).

Actually, given its constitutional limitations, the *Canada Health Act* is not really a health act but rather a spending act. It provides money in the national interest, but with conditions: the federal government must make available a Canada Health and Social Transfer to the provinces (the health part of which was worth $27 billion in 2011–12), and if provinces want their share they must establish a complying program for "insured health services and extended health care services" (section 4).

What, according to the act, are insured health services? The act specifies that they are physician services and outpatient and in-patient hospital services. In-patient hospital services include beds and the medical and nursing services and pharmaceuticals that patients require within hospital walls.

The *Canada Health Act* gives Canadians access to hospitals and physicians for the health services they need without any upfront payment. In addition, the act lays down five criteria that provinces must meet to be eligible for money transfers (section 7):

• public administration;
• comprehensiveness;
• universality;
• portability; and
• accessibility.

In other words, the provincial health funding plan must be managed by a public entity (such as a provincial ministry), it must provide all of the services required by the act, it must accept all patients, including those from other provinces, and everyone must have reasonable access to health care services.

Although the wording of the *Canada Health Act* is simple (the English version of the whole act is only around 4,000 words long), each of these criteria is contentious at times. That should not surprise us. In any human context, the more general the wording of an agreement, the likelier it is that disputes of interpretation will arise. Let's consider each of the criteria in turn.

Public Administration

This criterion only applies to the administration of the health plan – the plan must be publicly administered. However, and this is important, the *Canada Health Act* does not specifically lay down the requirement that hospitals must be administered publicly in a not-for-profit way. It also leaves open the door to other for-profit areas of health care. For instance, most Canadian physicians are in private practice and always have been. Furthermore, Canadians are likely to receive all kinds of diagnostic services (blood tests, X-rays, MRIs, etc.) in for-profit clinics. Opponents of privatization suggest that the existing privatization in these areas is inconsistent with the principles of medicare or the *Canada Health Act*. However, two fairly recent reports came to different conclusions.

The report of the Commission on the Future of Health Care in Canada, known as the Romanow report (2002), concluded that "Canadians view medicare as a moral enterprise, not a business venture," and Romanow argued for a limit on private provision: "At a minimum, I believe governments must draw a clear line between direct health services (such as hospital and medical care) and ancillary ones (such as food preparation and maintenance services). The former should be delivered primarily through our public, not-for-profit system, while the latter could be the domain of providers" (Romanow 2002, xxi).

The 2002 report of the Standing Senate Committee on Social Affairs, Science and Technology (the Kirby report) was more ambivalent. It left the door open to for-profit provision of direct health services; in other words, it was open to the possibility of for-profit hospitals and clinics (although for-profit service provision would be subject to the spirit of the *Canada Health Act*). We'll come back to this issue.

Comprehensiveness

Section 9 of the act states that "the health care insurance plan of a province must insure all insured health services provided by hospitals, medical practitioners or dentists" (the services dentists provide within hospital walls, that is). One group of writers (Forget et al. 2007, 19) thinks that this criterion should be deleted altogether: "the Canadian health care system is not now, never has been and should not even attempt to be all-encompassing. To retain the pretense of 'comprehensiveness' is to irresponsibly refuse to adjust citizens' expectations to the reality of government commitments."

They may have a point. Why provide services inside hospital walls you don't provide outside, like dental care? Moreover, no government can provide everything to everybody. Indeed, because the *Canada Health Act* only requires provinces to provide "necessary services," the comprehensiveness of medicare is already constrained. "Necessary" is not defined, and this opens the door to problems about boundary lines: services are either necessary or not. Cosmetic surgery is easily put in the "not necessary" column, but should reproductive health services be in it as well, or crucial counselling services? Opinions will vary. The ambivalent wording of this criterion requires professionals at all levels of health care to make decisions about what's necessary under the act and what's not, producing inconsistencies from location to location. Moreover, what constitutes a necessary service will change over time as well.

Universality

Universality means that all Canadians are in the same health care boat. Universality is the clearest expression of our care for others, whether we know them or not. The phrasing of the act encompasses all of us. Section 10 states that "the health care insurance plan of a province must entitle one hundred per cent of the insured persons of the province to the insured health services provided by the plan on uniform terms and conditions." One hundred per cent of us must be covered, rich and poor alike. We all have a vested interest in making sure the system works to provide high-quality care for every one of us.

Even though this clause (and others in the act) uses the word "insurance," it is insurance in only a technical sense, and this very universality belies the use of this term. Our neighbours down south face all kinds of problems associated with non-universality. For one thing, even after the passing of new health care legislation in the United States, tens of millions of ordinary folks have but limited access to health care. Insurance premiums are high. Prior condition exemptions limit protection in many policies, and US insurance companies routinely second guess (and disallow) decisions by physicians and hospitals. Insurance policies invariably are complex documents, written to protect the issuer more than the insured. By contrast, Canada has a single payer for all of us, namely the applicable provincial government, financed in part by federal transfer payments.

However, the above does not prevent some Canadians from advocating private funding to augment public funding for services covered under medicare, enabling, for instance, wealthier Canadians to bypass waiting lists. One problem with this is that the adoption of any such proposal would invariably weaken the universal commitment: if we're all in the same boat, we all want to make sure it doesn't leak. If we're in a yacht of our own, we tend not to look down to see how the canoes are faring.

Portability

No matter which province they come from, Canadians are free to travel the whole of our country and move from one province to another. The portability clause gives assurance that they may do so without jeopardizing their access to care, even though the details of health care provision are the exclusive domain of individual provinces. Section 11 of the act addresses this issue by stating that new residents must be provided with health care within three months and that a province's plan must cover care its residents receive in another province.

That last part is a bone of contention. Provinces set different rates of payment for services, and sometimes the differences are substantial. If you need medical care while you're on vacation or travelling for business, you may discover that the province of your residence does not pay anywhere near what you have to pay in the province in which you receive treatment, and you're out of pocket for the difference. It's up to the provinces to negotiate agreements to prevent Canadians from having to pay such expenses, and such agreements are in place for hospital services. However, agreements are not in place for all other types of services: for example, Quebec has a maximum daily rate for non-urgent treatments, and for physician services it pays only the lower of either the physician's fee or the Quebec rate for a similar service. In many cases Quebec residents need to pay for care directly and then apply for reimbursement themselves, whereas for residents of other provinces the physician simply bills the relevant provincial plan.

The portability criterion also applies to care received outside

Canada. However, conditions vary from country to country. In countries with medicare plans similar to ours (Australia, for instance), Canadians will receive emergency hospital services without upfront payment. Adrian and his wife were on a visit to the country of their birth when Johanna had an accident that required medical care. She had three visits to a local physician, a hospital visit, which included X-rays, and a consultation with a specialist. The total bill came to about $300 (and was covered by their travel insurance policy). By contrast, on a visit to the United States Adrian experienced a dangerously high pulse. Five hours in a hospital, a consultation with a cardiologist and a lung specialist, and a prescription for drugs cost their insurance company $15,000, and only part of that amount was reimbursed by their provincial health plan. Moreover, anything to do with Adrian's heart and lungs was excluded from his travel insurance policies for the next five years. Travelling in the United States may leave Canadians with a hefty bill for health care, as many have discovered. All Canadians should make sure they have a comprehensive travel health policy when they travel abroad, but especially in the United States. Travelling within Canada is far less scary. Even so, the *Canada Health Act* permits provinces to pay only the applicable provincial rate for care their residents receive in other provinces.

Accessibility

This criterion has two elements. The province:

- must provide patients with reasonable and not impeded access; and
- must provide reasonable compensation for physicians.

The key word in both clauses is "reasonable." The *Canada Health Act* in effect bars extra-billing, and it also does not permit charging more than a negotiated tariff or fee schedule. Ottawa wields as a stick the threat of reductions in transfer payments in response to non-compliance. But how is such a tariff or fee schedule set? Negotiations about physician fees, for instance, don't start with what individual physicians think they should get paid for specific services. Instead, a total for physician services is budgeted annually and then that pot of money is divided among physicians; in most cases the allocation for each physician is expressed in terms of specific fees for specific services. Other physicians, on salaries or alternative funding arrangements, also are paid out of this pot.

Different provinces have different rules about how physicians administratively participate in their health plans. They have a choice about whether or not to participate, but in most provinces it's an all-or-nothing choice: physicians must either opt into the plan (in which case they bill the plan for all services they provide to patients) or they must opt out (in which case they bill their patients for all services). These five *Canada Health Act* criteria are the framework within which provincial policies must ensure that no financial barrier exists at the point of service (physicians, hospitals). These criteria do not guarantee a problem-free medicare, as we shall see in subsequent chapters. Nevertheless, they have become so much a part of our Canadian identity that anyone proposing medicare reform seems compelled to respect them.

In summary, there are three main pegs on which to hang our thinking about medicare:

- Do all Canadians, poor and rich, have equal *access* to health care services?
- Are those services of sufficient *quality*, for the poor as well as the rich?
- How shall the system be *sustained*?

We'll come back more than once to this access-quality-sustainability chain.

By becoming acquainted with what the *Canada Health Act* requires, citizens will be more alert to what politicians may be saying as they seek votes. Is what the politicians say consistent with the *Canada Health Act*? Or is what they propose in conflict (hidden conflict perhaps) with any or all of the five criteria? We need to be citizen watchdogs especially at election time.

The 2004 Accord

In the past Canada's prime ministers have periodically sat down with provincial premiers to hammer out a new medicare agreement or accord. The federal government has focused on ensuring that provincial medicare policies continue to respect the five *Canada Health Act* principles. Provinces have bargained for more funds, taking into account contemporary health situations, such as the introduction of increasingly sophisticated and more costly equipment and procedures. The most recent agreement (2004) included the First Ministers' Accord on Health Care Renewal and the associated 10-Year Plan to Strengthen Health Care. However, the current federal government doesn't seem interested in convening such collective gatherings, on health care or on any other topic. Instead, the federal government has simply announced that it will continue the current level of funding plus 6% for two additional years past 2014, and then it will limit increases to the annual percentage gain in gross domestic product (GDP). It also seems to be far less interested than previous federal governments in what the provinces actually do with the funds and in enforcing the requirements of the *Canada Health Act*.

Canadian federalism is a balancing act between central and provincial jurisdictions. In domestic Canadian politics there is a perpetual tug-of-war with Ottawa on one side and various provincial and territorial capitals on the other (and the latter are not always of one mind). First ministers' meetings and debates may not seem all that gripping to most Canadians, but the resulting agreements have profound impacts. The 2004 medicare accord paid homage to the five principles of the *Canada Health Act*, while allowing for considerable provincial autonomy. The federal side tried to ensure that, for instance, a cancer patient receives the same level of care wherever he or she lives in Canada. However, the federal government acknowledged that health care is the responsibility of provincial and territorial governments, who have sole jurisdiction over health care provision within their own borders. Some provinces (think of Prince Edward Island, for instance) simply lack the means to offer services that larger and richer provinces may be able to afford, and thus they need extra funds. That is a reality of Canadian domestic politics.

Canada faces an added complication. Setting federal standards for services of any kind presumes the existence of a national will. But at minimum Canada has two national wills, one residing in Quebec, as its leaders keep asserting, and the other in the rest of the country. Any claims of a national will are interpreted in Quebec as being the will of English Canada. In addition, people in western Canada sometimes look askance at those who live in the East, and so on. All federal-provincial agreements need to respect this federation reality. Ottawa does have an array of instruments to entice (even compel) provinces to adhere to national standards. It can regulate the flow of funds, not only in general but also in targeted ways. It can provide expertise. It can hold provinces to account by threatening to withhold funds.

So, given all these complications, what did the 2004 accord achieve?

- It settled on a pool of funds flowing from Ottawa to the provinces, adjusting for the economic character of individual provinces.

- It guaranteed an annual 6% increase in funds to the provinces.
- It established national goals for waiting time, with provinces identifying their own improvement priorities.
- Ottawa provided a federal advisor on wait times.
- The accord provided stability for ten years.

What will happen after 2014, when it appears that the federal government will be less of a watchdog overseeing whether the provinces live up to the criteria of the *Canada Health Act*? That is the big question, and every Canadian has an interest in the answer. Will the apparent weakening of the federal government's watchdog function result in greater variations in health care, with richer provinces providing more comprehensive health care to their residents than poorer ones? Will the lessening presence of "Ottawa" drive us to feel ourselves more "East Coast" or "Prairie"? Will our sense of national social citizenship weaken in the coming years? These are troubling questions that have always been present, but they will perhaps produce greater tension in the coming years.

Provincial Government Funding

We have seen that the combination of the *Canada Health Act* and the 2004 accord between Ottawa and the provinces provided a direction (the five principles) and a broad federal-provincial funding agreement. However, neither principles nor periodic agreements settle disputes forever. There will always be plenty of claiming and posturing. The central problem doesn't go away: provinces need to provide within their own jurisdiction what we have agreed upon as a nation (or two): reliable, accessible, and equitable medicare for all Canadians. It is time to have a preliminary look at how the provinces actually deliver the health care that we look for in our own communities when we need a physician or a hospital. Who actually provides the money for total medicare expenses?

- Roughly 65% comes from provincial health care budgets.
- Roughly 30% comes out of citizens' pockets (directly or through employer or private insurance policies).
- About 5% is derived from other government sources.

Of that 30% private funding, roughly 34% is spent on medications, 23% on dental services, and 18% on upgrading hospital services (from a ward to semi-private room, for instance).

Now let's have a look at per capita spending province by province, using 2010 figures. (In our discussion we'll leave aside the Yukon, Northwest Territories, and Nunavut: their sparse populations settled in huge territories present special funding problems.)

Figure 1.1 shows that there is a significant variation in total per capita spending, ranging from an Alberta high of $6,864 per citizen down to a Quebec low of $4,966. Provincial treasury spending follows the same pattern (Alberta high at $4,704, Quebec low at $3,255).

Private sector contributions (from citizens' pockets or through insurance company policies) also vary from province to province. They are highest in Ontario, where they represent well above 30% of total spending, whereas they are substantially lower in Newfoundland and Labrador (22%), Saskatchewan (23%), and Manitoba (24%). One would expect that higher per capita spending would produce better access to and quality of medical care. But this isn't necessarily so. A 2011 analysis of Alberta's high per capita spending yielded no evidence that the province was also leading the nation in terms of access and quality of care.

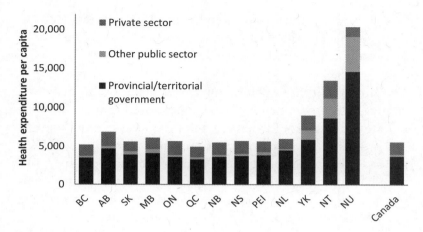

Figure 1.1: Per capita health expenditure (age and sex adjusted) by province/territory, by source of funds, 2010

Provincial governments spend a lot of health care money on their citizens. On the one hand, survey after survey shows that Canadians like their medicare, describing it with words like "iconic" and the phrase "the country's most cherished social program." At the same time, many Canadians are critical of the way it operates. Medicare funds hospitals and physicians but does not cover all aspects of health care, which is why about 30% of funding comes out of our pockets, directly or by way of insurance policies. Dental services and drugs (with some exceptions) are the big exclusions. Canadians are also critical of the services that are provided. In international surveys that spanned the years 1998 to 2010, Canadians were asked to assess their medicare. Here are the results:

- On the average, roughly one third of Canadians surveyed indicated that only minor changes to the system were necessary.

- Up to two thirds indicated the need for a fundamental change (10–15% of these respondents said that a complete rebuild was needed).

The surveys did not explore what was meant by fundamental change. Some commentators have proposed that the level of private funding should increase, but the surveys do not address this proposal. They do point to Canadians' dissatisfaction with the long waits at almost every point of the care journey and with having to pay a lot of money for drugs. Although a commitment to improving access was part of the 2004 accord, the results that have been achieved seem inadequate.

The *Canada Health Act*, vague though it is, represents the heart of our medicare and it's not up for debate. Its principles have been supported by Canadians for more than half a century. Provincial funding and the provision of services are under constant review. The way in which these components combine in years to come will determine the future shape of Canada's medicare system. Now is the time for all Canadians to let their legislators (federal and provincial) know that we need to keep, and improve, medicare. Some politicians and pundits exhibit a weak commitment to our medicare, expressing doubts about sustainability and citing demographics, aging, and the seemingly out-of-control costs. In the next chapter we'll lay out the case for sustainability, taking these factors into account. However, we'll also point out that changes are needed to medicare, and we'll describe these changes in subsequent chapters.

A tip for you:
Ask candidates at the next federal or provincial election (or your current representatives, if they have a "listening tour") for their thoughts about medicare. Do they think it is sustainable? If not, what are their plans?

CHAPTER 2

Is Medicare Sustainable?

Here is what we have in mind when we contemplate the sustainability of medicare. Can Canadians continue to count on the tradition, now more than a half-century old, that their fellow citizens will help them to avoid the serious financial calamities that might result from illness and accidents? Moreover, can we enable health care professionals to help us cope well with the impact of chronic diseases and aging? Or will economic, demographic, fiscal, and financial forces overwhelm our commitments? Our answer to the first two questions is a resounding yes and to the third question a well-considered no. We tackle the third question in this chapter and the next one.

Is medicare sustainable? Politicians, journalists, economists, and academics ask this question regularly, and it makes frequent appearances in letters to the editor. The question expresses our national anxiety. Some answer yes, some answer no. Both answers have consequences. Many Canadians worry that if medicare is not sustainable the responsibility for paying the high cost of medical services will once again fall upon the shoulders of individuals and families. Most middle-class and working-class families already stoop under the burdens of their daily household expenses. Many Canadians carry dangerously high debt loads. Consider the effect of adding medical costs of roughly $4,000 per person each year to an average Canadian household budget (this figure approximates current per capita provincial spending on health care). That's about $16,000 per year for an average Canadian family. A quick glance at the costs of private insurance policies in the United States will confirm that private insurance won't alleviate the problem. If medicare cannot be sustained, the consequences are unthinkable. Even the possibility of a dramatically slimmed down medicare is worrisome.

What will it take to sustain medicare? Setting ever higher taxes? Providing fewer health care services? Providing less access? Keeping medicare but putting the squeeze on other public services, such as education?

This book demonstrates that these questions need not keep us awake at night with worry. Is medicare sustainable? We answer this key question with a resounding yes. We will argue in the next chapter that it can be sustained without dramatically higher taxes, but changes will need to be made soon. In this chapter we will first consider, and refute, some of the "no" answers. We will examine three sets of buzzwords that are often brought into play: aging population, inadequate tax base, and runaway costs.

Aging Population: Are We Facing a Coming Avalanche or Tsunami?

Older people use medicare more than younger folks. We hear warnings that disaster is at hand because Canada is aging: the boomers are coming, the boomers are coming! Is that conclusion warranted, or is it mere fear mongering by people who may have a political or ideological axe to grind? Let's look at the facts.

It's true that Canada is aging. This demographic development is often assessed by calculating the dependency ratio, which expresses the proportion of people over 65 plus children below 15 as compared with everyone else. In other words, it's a measure of dependents compared with earners. If there are more dependents than earners, the social costs of larger numbers of people will have to be met by smaller numbers, and the economy comes under stress. In many developed countries, especially in Western Europe, where both rates have been low for years and immigration is restricted, the number of dependents has already become substantially larger than the number of earners. Fortunately, Canada is in a much better position. Although our current birth rate will not produce a steadily growing population, our yearly high immigrant influx will more than compensate. The good news is that in Canada the Index 1 line (50% workers, 50% dependents) will not be crossed until at least 2016, and the subsequent adverse change in the ratio will be slower than in other countries. Demographically, we are not facing an avalanche but a glacier, not a tsunami but a manageable tide. The 2011 census should comfort us all. Since 2005 our population has grown from 31.6 million to 33.5 million, an increase of 5.9%, the highest increase of all G8 nations, and our current immigration policy favours individuals who will have a positive impact on the economy.

Canada is indeed aging, but the inference that therefore we shall have to face a disproportional increase in health care spending (and that health care costs will consume an ever larger portion of the gross domestic product or GDP) is mere speculation. The facts don't bear out the intuition, as a number of economists and other observers are saying.

Consider this also. From 1921 to 2001, years in which life expectancy increased dramatically, for every increase of 1% in life expectancy, the economy as a whole gained 9.6 % in national GDP and 6.7% in per capita GDP. In other words, the economy as a whole grew much faster than the population. Of course, with the help of technology (e.g., computers) productivity increased dramatically in those years, substantially improving our GDP. But we must not overlook the fact that in those years people came to live longer and thus contributed much longer to the workforce with their experience and skills, which are important components of productivity. These statistics indicate that aging adds to, not subtracts from, the GDP. In addition, while it is true that for a number of years many Canadians have retired before they turned 65, that trend seems to be reversing, as people in good health work beyond that age. Government policies as well as personal preferences will play a role. At minimum these trends raise the prospect that even though older people use medicare more than younger folks, their usage will not break the bank. The impact will be just a fraction each year, easily manageable.

Moreover, older people are living longer because they are healthier. It is highly likely that a 75-year-old some years from now won't need as much health care as a 75-year-old today. Even a modest reduction in the kind of chronic ailments that often manifest themselves in seniors will yield a substantial reduction in health care costs. Some chronic illnesses may be reduced in quantity and severity by campaigns aimed at healthy living. The great motivator will be the fact that better health will make life more pleasant for seniors. As a consequence the pressure on medicare will lessen.

Knowledgeable commentators point to the fact that substantial health care expenditures occur in the last few years of life, a relatively short period in an individual's lifespan. It won't do to predict health care costs simply by counting years from birth, as many do (e.g., "everyone over 65"). We can more accurately predict health care expenditures for seniors by taking into account years left until death. Not everyone over 65 is draining health care coffers. Two commentators even demonstrated that when proximity to death is taken into account, there is a negative relationship between overall aging and health care expenditures (but the difference is so slight that we don't want to stress this finding).

Other studies should also lessen our anxiety about health care costs for aging. The Canadian Health Services Research Foundation maintains that health care expenditures for seniors will increase roughly 1% per year until 2030, less than projected growth in GDP. A second study demonstrated that in four Canadian provinces an increase in the proportion of older people was actually associated with a decrease in health care costs. A third study concluded that older folks will have far less mobility issues than generations past, an indication of improved health. There is a plethora of other studies with similar findings. One using data from developed countries concluded that over the years 1960–2000 health care spending on seniors had increased no more than 8.8% in the "worst" of those countries; the average was well below 1% per year. This study included European countries with an already unfavourable dependency ratio.

Here is a summary of many studies on this topic: "The reality, as reflected in a steadily accumulating collection of research studies, is that to date the effects of aging per se on health care costs have been quite limited ... Projections suggest that future effects, while not inconsequential, will appear gradually, and will be within the capacity of historical rates of economic growth" (Barer et al. 1995). In other words, we are not facing an avalanche, and we are not facing a tsunami. The impact of aging on costs is more like a slowly moving glacier. Increasing costs because of aging can be absorbed as part of the normal development and innovation of the health care system and will be less than growths in GDP.

This is not to say that we should ignore the effects of aging. Statistics Canada predicts that our population over age 65 will double between 2011 and 2036, with the number of upper seniors (those over 85) increasing from 675,000 to 1,700,000 (a 150% increase). Even if the current over 60 group enjoys better health at age 85 than the current over 85 cohort, the costs will indeed rise. However, when experts plot those cost expectations over the time frame indicated, we're talking about at worst a 2% impact per year, which is not only less than dramatic, but manageable with proper policies. Those policy responses should take into account both structural innovations and improvements in efficiency, as we shall see in subsequent chapters.

Do We Have a Large Enough Tax Base?

Even if we do not need to lie awake with worries about the impact on medicare expenditures of aging per se given even modest increases in GDP, some will still be concerned about the prospect of a shrinking tax base, seeing that the proportion of workers will decrease.

Let's have another look at that dependency ratio. What have Canadians over age 65 got in common with those under 15? Both groups are supported, the latter by parents and the former by the whole of society through income support, mainly through the Canada Pension Plan and Old Age Security. Both groups have access to publicly funded health care. In other words, people at both ends of the demographic spectrum are dependent on the taxpaying population of working-age Canadians. Although Canada is in far better shape than, for instance, European countries, it is true that Statistics Canada projects the proportion of dependents (over 65 and under 15) to increase between 2011 and 2036 from 45% to 65%, with most of that increase the result of the over 65 group increasing from roughly 20% to just under 40% of our total population.

Some worried people easily slide into using the term "dependency burden," a term of resentment if not dismissal. However, research data indicate that they should refrain from using this vocabulary: just as current morbidity patterns do not predict future ones, the dependency ratio may not provide a reliable predictor for years hence. The current percentage of people over 65 plus those under 15 is not a reliable predictor of the taxpaying or working population. Current trends already show increasing numbers of people working well past 65, and the proportion of working women is still increasing.

Moreover, the dependency ratio is clearly amenable to policy intervention. For instance, governments might enact policies that encourage people to remain in the workforce longer, as some countries have already done. In early 2012 our federal government announced that it will seek to move the age at which Canadians begin to receive the universal Old Age Security benefit from 65 to 67. Many workers may want to work longer anyway, for financial reasons and reasons of interest, health, and energy. Some recent voices argue that we should encourage even more immigration, jumping to 400,000 or more newcomers yearly. Those measures and decisions together would produce more taxable income.

Runaway Costs?

We have ruled out aging per se as a substantial contributor to growth in health care expenditures. However, it cannot be denied that for awhile now costs have increased faster than rates of inflation. Contributing factors are the introduction of ever more expensive pharmaceuticals and technologies, coupled with the increased prevalence of chronic conditions such as obesity, heart disease, and diabetes. We should be concerned.

In wealthy nations health care expenditures are taking an increasing share of GDP, and Canada is no exception. Economists have a term for those goods and services for which demand grows faster than income: they call them "luxury goods." Surely health care is not a luxury. No individual or family faced with a serious illness would call it that. Moreover, in health care we are not dealing with an excess of demand over income but rather a disproportional rise in expenditures. That suggests that provincial governments and health care leaders should focus on improving efficiency and productivity and containing

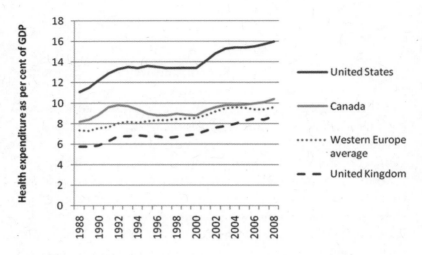

Figure 2.1: Trends in health expenditure as a share of gross domestic product, selected countries, 1988–2008

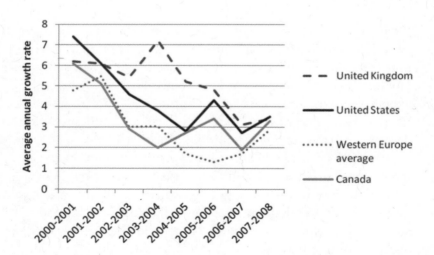

Figure 2.2: Average annual growth rate in public health expenditure, selected countries, 2000–2008

the fees paid to health care providers. As we shall demonstrate in subsequent chapters, there is lots of potential for substantial cost savings.

Canada's health expenditure patterns are similar to those of other developed countries. Figure 2.1 illustrates the trends.

The United States tops the list in almost every comparative study of health care expenditures. Canada, the United Kingdom, and western European countries report very similar expenditure levels as a percentage of GDP. Although Canada showed a bit of a bulge in the early 1990s and is still a comparatively high spender, it seems that our pattern of expenditure levels is generally akin to those of the United Kingdom and western European countries.

The United States also is an exception in terms of public expenditure as a percentage of total health care spending, with 47%. Canada's public share is 71%, that of the United Kingdom is just over 82%, and that of the rest of Western Europe is roughly 76%. Other countries seem to be facing the same challenges that we are facing.

Figure 2.2 illustrates the annual growth rate in public health care expenditures for the same geographical areas. It shows that public spending is not a runaway monster, as some commentators might make you think. In fact, the growth in public spending has been trending downward since the beginning of this millennium.

That we see the same pattern in various areas of the world should not surprise us. Policy ideas, clinical techniques, pharmaceuticals, and equipment quickly migrate from one country to another within the global economy, through both official and unofficial channels. Not all countries included in these graphs have a similar health care system, but the differences need not concern us here. In spite of the differences, total spending patterns are very similar.

We have looked at the effects of aging, tax-base develop-ments, and comparative trends in health care spending and concluded that none of these factors is a major threat to the sus-tainability of medicare. Talk of a health care crisis has no basis in reality. When you hear politicians and ideology-inspired pun-dits make claims about the viability of our medicare (or lack of it), citing any one of these areas, challenge them if you are able. Research is clear: demographics (aging) is not a fatal threat, not in actual costs nor with respect to a diminishing tax base. Policies can be put in place that will better control health care spending, and thus concerns about ever higher costs outstrip-ping the increases in our GDP can be addressed. In subsequent chapters we will talk about primary care clinics, an overdue Pharmacare program, a much more sensible approach to caring for seniors, and about ill health prevention. We also think that hospital costs can be pushed back.

A tip for you:
When a public figure talks about the tsunami of an aging population, ask them what impact aging will have on costs next year. (The answer should be that the effects of an aging population will increase health care expenditures by something less than 2%.) Ask them why they think we can't cope with that small a change. Hold them to account for their scaremongering.

CHAPTER 3

Medicare and Not Much Else?

In chapter 2 we addressed three economic challenges to the sustainability of our medicare that are regularly advanced in the media or in political speeches. We looked at the buzzwords used by those who feel that our medicare is unsustainable, in part or in whole: aging population; inadequate tax base; runaway costs. Although action is required to address all three situations, the evidence shows that Canadians can rest assured that our medicare can be sustained.

However, sustaining medicare will require that steps be taken now to address emerging health issues. It is not particularly budget and taxation steps that are needed, but rather measures that will ensure better health and health care for all citizens. The latter is not rocket science. We know, for instance, that proper care for expecting mothers and proper early childhood nutrition and activities have permanent positive effects on personal health and produce positive economic returns. Moreover, it is often cheaper to invest in eliminating poverty than it is to merely treat its symptoms, and those symptoms include ill health. The actions we take today will have long-reaching consequences for individuals, for our health care system, and for the whole of Canadian society. Inaction, too, will have consequences. If we pay less attention to health care and ill health prevention there will be greater losses in the long run.

More ill health will negatively affect the economy. Proper investment pays off.

While actions must be taken now, these need not touch the core elements of our medicare. There is no need to dramatically increase private funding. There is no need to change the five criteria of the *Canada Health Act*. There is no need to play with access-quality-sustainability trade-offs: all three are achievable. Taking action means investing money, but investing wisely with a view to achieving social efficiency. Spending smarter will be the theme of subsequent chapters.

However, before we discuss various areas that are ripe for improvement, we need to face a fourth challenge. It has to do with medicare's financial sustainability. Financial sustainability is different from economic sustainability. Economic sustainability has to do with making good investments in health care so that the returns in better health are worth the costs. Financial sustainability has to do with the amount of money that is available to pay for health care and the percentages of budgets that are consumed by health care spending. Here's an example of the difference between economic and financial sustainability. A company can be utterly efficient and have a product the market wants (i.e., it is economically sustainable), and yet it can go out of business when it runs out of capital to pay its workers' salaries, the rent and power bills for its office space, and so on (i.e., it is not financially sustainable). It runs out of capital when shareholders don't want to buy more shares or the banks don't want to lend it more money, for whatever reasons.

Medicare's financial sustainability is a political and not an economic focus. Those who focus on the financial sustainability of medicare weigh what level of health care spending Ottawa and the provinces can afford given a presumed maximum level of taxation. No matter how efficient the system and sound its economics, it isn't financially sustainable if there isn't enough money to maintain it. Ontario's premier, Dalton McGuinty, produced the most direct and brutal expression of this point of view: "At these rates [of increase], there will come a time when the ministry of health is the only ministry we can afford to have and we still won't be able to afford the ministry of health." While few repeat McGuinty's hyperbole, some share his point of view by claiming that increases in provincial health care spending are crowding out spending in other important social areas, such as education. Indeed, it cannot be denied that per capita provincial spending on health care is taking up an increasing share of provincial budgets. It is also consuming an increasing share of provincial gross domestic products (GDPs), with one observer predicting a rise from 7.7% in 2008 to 13.1% in 2035.

So let's first have a look at whether recent provincial government budgets provide evidence that other essential services are being squeezed by ever larger health care slices of the revenue pie. For instance, are education budgets declining, something we might expect given that birth rates and school populations are declining? One observer undertook a major study to find the answer and concluded that "the statistical evidence ... provides no support for the hypothesis that, during the sample period [1988–2004], health care expenditures crowded out either non-health provincial program spending in aggregate or any major category of provincial government spending. Indeed, the results imply the opposite – that health and non-health expenditures tend to move in tandem" (Landon et al. 2006).

What we need to understand is this: setting a budget is a political act, and politics is about making choices. Each provincial government sets its own budget priorities under the influence of many factors (political philosophy, public opinion and confidence, lobbying pressures, perceived needs, etc.).

Political choices determine the size of government and the size of the tax base to support public services. There are no inevitabilities. Different political parties (and commentators) set different priorities with respect to the type and extent of services that should be provided and have different opinions about what tax rates are desirable. These choices are driven by political convictions as well as by financial and economic factors. Those who favour small governments and low taxes will want to increase private funding of health care, but their position (health care funding is financially unsustainable) will be defended on ideological and not financial grounds.

Will things be disastrous in years to come? We do not think so. We will argue in the following chapters that governments can act with skill and acumen to halt trends toward ever increasing costs, with policies that work. At a minimum, they can take steps to slow unwanted trends sufficiently to ensure a secure future for medicare.

Taxes

We also need to think a bit more about the nature of taxes. Right-wing politicians (more so in the United States than in Canada) have convinced a lot of voters that taxes are bad in principle, especially taxes to be paid by the rich. Taxes take money out of citizens' pockets; leaving the money in those pockets stimulates the economy because citizens are able to buy more goods and services. Lower taxes will boost the economy and eventually eliminate the gaps between government incomes and expenses (deficits), or so is the claim. But is it really that simple? The massive deficits and sluggish economy in the United States would suggest otherwise, and many economists don't buy this argument either.

We (the authors) don't think that taxes are bad in principle. Taxes provide the public services we all use every day: the roads, the schools, the buses, and clean water. Designated taxes support efforts to keep the air we breathe clean and prosecute polluters. We may not always agree about specific government policies and actions that produce particular rates, amounts, and types of taxes, but we rarely disagree about the need for taxes per se.

We both object to the blatant attempts of most governments to have us think that they do us favours. Think of the large billboards in which governments take credit for providing new highways or upgrades, often with the names of premiers and transportation ministers prominently displayed as if they personally are the givers of good gifts. Government is neither a parent nor a philanthropist. It is a body entrusted with resources and charged with the responsibility to use these wisely for the common good in just ways. Taxes are valuable resources. Taxes are parts of our incomes reserved for the common good. Taxes belong to civil society. In a truly civil society we strive for justice for all and always have our neighbours in mind. Taxes are not a plot to relieve us by force (law) of what is our own but rather they are our contributions to the maintenance of a vital and just state. As we ought to be happy when we can give gifts to our families, so we should be pleased when our taxes enable good things to happen to our fellow Canadians.

Here is Adrian's story.

As an immigrant I do not object to paying taxes. In March 1954 I came to Canada at age nineteen with $30 in my pocket and my few material possessions in a canvas army bag. Taxes (both from my country of origin and from Canada) had paid for my journey across the Atlantic and the long train ride from Halifax to Toronto. Canada had a job for me, and I began paying taxes immediately. In the fall of 1955 I decided to enroll in McMaster University. For three years the federal government supported my university attendance with tax dollars, as the cost of educating me was more than the fees I paid. I also received scholarships and bursaries, some from federal and provincial governments. In 1958 I graduated, and until my retirement in 1994 I worked for a living and paid taxes: income tax, sales taxes, import duties, gasoline taxes, real estate taxes, and so on. As a worker and citizen I used Canada's roads, its airports, and its libraries, and I felt protected by its army, its police, and its firefighters. I always tried to not pay any more than the law required, but I never grumbled about the legitimate amount. How could I? As this country had invited me in and enabled me to not only find my economic way but also enjoy its people and its features, how could I not help create conditions for others to experience the same? This is just one example of contributing to the common good.

There are times when taxes are bad. Individual and corporate dictators and tyrants see taxes as an opportunity to enrich themselves, not as instruments to bless the lives of their citizens. Over the centuries, as life became more complex, the state more powerful and expansive, and trade more global, taxes increased in size and number. Part of human history is economic history, and part of economic history is the growth in the complexity of life and the parallel development of taxation. Governments of all shapes and sizes have found numerous ways of getting money from ordinary citizens, for both good and bad purposes. Some governments have been brutal in their demands; others have tried to tax their citizens no more than was necessary. In a time when the church hierarchy was as much a civil as an ecclesiastical body, one Pope levied a heavy tax on windmills: he said that the wind was a gift of God to the church, so as God's representative on earth the church was entitled to part of the proceeds of that gift.

Yes, there is plenty to gripe about when it comes to taxes. The folly of World War I produced deep economic misery for all of Europe and beyond. At present, the Iraqi and Afghani conflicts combined with the unbridled Wall Street greed that permeates the US financial system are a major threat to the US economy and the economies of other nations. Western nations are now carrying enormous public debts, partly because of misguided policies. Those debts will produce heavy tax burdens for our children and their children. Governments, like all large institutions, inevitably produce much waste and require money to be spent on items with which we disagree. Elected officials and bureaucrats are not always honest as they use their positions and power to enrich themselves.

Yet we must not let governmental folly mask the essence of taxation. Taxes are the moneys we raise collectively to enable governments to have us jointly bear common burdens. Deep inside, we all know that. Ask people who grumble about taxes which parts of governments they would do without, and their answers will be vague.

Table 3.1 (next page), for example, shows part of the 2009 Edmonton city municipal budget. The main services that have a direct beneficial impact comprise 16.8% of the $2.066 billion budget.

Edmonton citizens work together to fund these benefits. We haven't even counted such things as street and road construction and repair, snow cleaning, sewer services, water services, garbage collection, control over the way homes and other buildings are constructed, and public transit.

The story of provincial government budgets is the same in principle. Table 3.2 (next page), for example, shows a summary of some of the areas in which the Alberta government spent money in 2009.

Expenditures in these eight areas take up 81.6% of all provincial tax revenues, which are made up of the money collected through many kinds of provincial taxation and the money received from the federal government through transfer payments. This is a massive amount of money, some spent for the benefit of all (e.g., health, transportation, education services),

Table 3.1 From Edmonton 2009 municipal budget

Neighbourhood and community development	$51 million	2.4%
Recreation facilities	$63 million	3.1%
Emergency medical services	$10 million	0.4%
Fire rescue services	$140 million	6.8%
Parks	$45 million	2.2%
Libraries	$40 million	1.9%

Table 3.2 From Alberta 2009 budget

Advanced education and technology	8.6% of all spending
Education	16.9%
Seniors and community support	5.4%
Children and youth services	3.1%
Agriculture and rural development	3.1%
Transportation	6.1%
Employment and immigration	2.8%
Health and wellness	35.6%

some for the benefit of some (e.g., services for seniors). Indeed, some of the money gets spent for the benefit of those who suffer and have difficulty living a full citizen life (e.g., employment and immigration services for people with mental illness and other serious social and economic problems). We should be glad that we are collectively able to create the conditions of a modern state in which potentially all of us can thrive. We're talking about elementary justice.

Of course, not all that money ends up in the hands of those who need it. Bureaucracy gobbles up a substantial proportion of it.

However, no state can operate without a bureaucracy. Justice requires that for the money to be well spent we need checks and balances, laws and regulations, and administration and control.

The services that the federal government provides for our federal tax dollars seem to be farther removed from our daily life than the services provided by provincial and municipal governments: the federal government funds our military, legal systems, diplomacy, international relationships, treaties, and sophisticated economic measures (e.g., Bank of Canada). However, even some of the federal budget relates directly to services for the needy among us. International aid (spending in this area is pitifully low in Canada, alas) and employment insurance are but two elements that deserve attention. Moreover, fiscal (taxation) policy is often used to stimulate sectors in the economy that need temporary help, such as strategic boosts in employment.

Each June or July, newspapers usually publish a public notice from the Vancouver-based Fraser Institute, a conservative think tank. It gives us a date on which the average Canadian can begin to pocket his or her earnings. The claim is that up to that point the monetary rewards of labour have gone to various governments. The public notice bemoans the fact that we spend much of the year sending our wages to our governments. But why? Has there been no benefit to the average Canadian from his or her contribution to public services? Why not take pride in the fact that we willingly share whatever level of our wealth we earn through our labour with our fellow citizens through the properties we own together, such as roads, airports, and municipal services like water and sewage services, garbage collection, recycling depots, parks, trails, and festivities? We help those Canadians who can't help themselves: the sick, the mentally ill, the aged, the handicapped, and so on.

In line with our general views on taxes, we believe that governments should consider revenue strategies to meet future

increases in health expenditure so that medicare can be sustained. Some taxes (e.g., taxes on natural resource revenues and
corporate taxes) elicit a smaller negative reaction from voters at
election time. To make tax increases more palatable, politicians should remind Canadians regularly that our medicare is
a commitment to one another for sharing the financial burden
of illness. Some years ago the Alberta government folded health
care "premiums" into general taxation. The result of that political decision is that Alberta citizens are no longer reminded of
this commitment by contributing a monthly premium to the
notion of sharing, and we all get lulled into thinking that medicare is a favour provided by governments that is somehow free.
It's not. Medicare is all of us putting money in a pot from which
we can draw when we need it.

Responding to the Challenges: Some Principles

We are convinced that taxes are a positive contribution to a civil
and also compassionate society. We are also convinced that governments should do everything in their power to ensure that
taxes are well spent. With respect to our medicare, this means
that government policies should be designed to ensure that health
care is provided efficiently and in a fiscally responsible manner
and that the health care system produces the good health impacts
it is expected to provide.

Improving Efficiency

Few would argue with the notion of improving efficiency, but
what exactly is efficiency? It is not the same as cutting budgets.
What we want in health care is a positive return on investment,
with "return" meaning health first, not dollars first. As one slo-
gan has it, we want to add years to life and life to years.

Investing is not a one-time event. The health care system is dynamic, ever-changing, and experiencing new pressures requiring new responses. We need to entertain multiple strategies that are reviewed continuously. Is this or that program effective? Does it provide proper care (with the emphasis on care)? Can we eliminate ineffective programs, thereby freeing up money for better ones?

Expenditures need to be managed well, and this is not a simple task. For instance, health care is labour intensive. Health care money spent by users is also income for providers. Perhaps users want to pay less and providers want to receive more. Those different desires can lead to opposing strategies and tension, as a number of researchers have pointed out. Users may want to limit the income of providers (hospitals and medical practitioners), and providers may want to have users (taxpayers or patients who contribute) pay more.

If we focus on health care cost control, we need to look at two major factors:

1 What is the cost of each treatment?
2 How many treatments are necessary?

To find out what we spend in total, we multiply cost and volume. To reduce our total spending, we need to change either one of the two or both.

This is not a simple matter. Say we restrict the per consultation fee paid to doctors (cost), thereby reducing their incomes. It is likely that physicians will then want to see more patients (volume), which may not be a good thing for our health. Good diagnosis depends on sound interaction between physician and patient, and sound interactions take time, both for conversation and for more or less technical assessments (measuring blood pressure, listening to the heart, etc.). Conversation as part of physician consultations is under stress, as one physician argued on a CBC radio program. He lamented the fact that under the pressure of full waiting rooms, family physicians are losing their diagnostic skill, which requires that they take the time to simply observe and carefully listen to their patients. Instead, they quickly write referrals and prescribe a battery of (often expensive) tests.

When we look at the extensive literature on the relationship between expenditure and actual health outcomes, we discover a very weak link between the two. Simply spending more and doing more health care things won't necessarily improve our health. We need to take into account social efficiency in health care, which means making the right investments to achieve better health.

A Proposed Direction

We have already argued that the impact of aging on the future of our medicare is not an avalanche but a glacier. This means that we have time to make incremental changes; dramatic ones are not needed. (Dramatic changes often prove to be counterproductive.) What should those changes be?

Here is how we see the objective of a reformed Canadian health care system: *The right person enables the right care in the right setting, on time, every time.* Every single one of those words is important.

Right person. Each health care worker works at what he or she is trained to do. Physicians do what physicians should do, as do registered nurses, and so on. This produces job satisfaction as well as economic benefits.

Enables. Each person must enable the right care, not merely provide it. Given that our medicare system will be more and more concerned with chronic diseases in the future, it is important to keep in mind that patients are important partners in care. They need to be informed about their condition and knowledgeable about prognosis and course of action. The role of the health care provider is that of enabler of care, supporting patients in managing their own care and supporting patients' families and friends who provide care.

Right care. It is true that knowledge of the right care (e.g., knowledge coming from new research) takes a long time to be widely implemented. We need to take steps to identify best care practices and shorten implementation time.

Right setting. High-volume settings tend to produce better clinical outcomes. However, for facilities to carry out high volumes of care we have to have a smaller number of larger institutions, and this often imposes hardship on patients and their families, especially seniors, who must travel to one of these high-volume settings to get the care they need and experience dislocation. Many argue the benefit of the least restrictive alternative, meaning an emphasis on maintaining a patient's independence and keeping them in familiar surroundings for as long as possible, using home care, telephone consults, and community settings (clinics).

On time. The phrasing of the *Canadian Health Act* criterion of reasonable access explicitly addresses financial access, but long waits also impede access. Although some progress has been made since the 2004 accord in reducing wait times, the system has a long way to go.

Every time. We mean consistent care, in which providers learn from their mistakes and provide good care for everybody.

Canadian medicare reform is not simply a matter of more money, whether from federal transfers or private funding. As we have argued and now stress again, it is a long-term matter of the right person enabling the right care in the right setting, on time and every time. It is about improved efficiency, both technical and social. It's about making changes in every province, with every health service, and at every point in the health care continuum. The rest of this book will elaborate these points.

Values

Before we get into the changes to medicare that we think are needed in the following chapters, it bears repeating that any changes should be consistent with the enduring values of Canadian health care. We owe it to previous generations, and to our children and grandchildren, to maintain the basic trust Canadians have in our medicare. Strategies to control health care costs interact with other values, such as equity. For instance, requiring consumer co-payments will have a disproportionate impact on the lives of the poor.

We strongly believe that reform strategies should be shaped by the values we share and by the interest of both users and providers. Here is our list of concerns.

- *Reform strategies should express concern for disadvantaged populations and address as-yet-unmet needs.* Health needs are unevenly distributed in the population; they vary by age, location, employment status, and other factors such as belonging to a First Nation. To what extent should policies focus on improving the health status of the disadvantaged versus being targeted at majority populations? What is the right mix of interventions to be funded?
- *Reform strategies should emphasize the least restrictive alternative.* System design should recognize the importance of patient independence, even in seniors' accommodation.
- *The three value perspectives should be weighed: the patient, clinician, and economic perspectives.* Patients

want to be treated with dignity and have speedy access, good facilities, and excellent care, but judgments about proper procedures are in the hands of clinicians. Clinicians must work within an economic framework, which is in the hands of administrators. These three perspectives, namely the perspectives of the patient, clinician, and administrator, are all important, and weighing them together is an important part of health care.

- *Economic incentives should be used as appropriate.* Economic incentives have a proper place in shaping system development, and we'll explore how these might play a role in health care.
- *Different provider forms should be explored.* Is there a care role for for-profit providers (excluding professional corporations)? Are there reasons for distinguishing between small and large corporations?

This list highlights the rich number of factors that have an impact on system design and management of the system. Moreover, our health care system is ever changing, and there will never be a shortage of moments of decision.

Choices about the future of health care involve trade-offs and tensions across a range of dimensions. The most obvious tensions are often the economic ones, but other tensions are equally vital: centralized versus decentralized; research evidence versus long experience; large, remote institutions versus small, near institutions; and primary care versus chronic care.

Newspapers and magazines regularly feature medicare items. Most often these revolve around easy solutions and some simplistic recommendation (e.g., pay a small fee for every doctor's visit). However, medicare is complex, and each solution has effects throughout the system. We hope that this book will contribute to a realistic view of medicare by Canadians.

Our next task is to outline proposals for desirable changes and point to the investments required to improve, protect, and preserve Canada's medicare.

> *A tip for you:*
> Ask your friends about taxes. Do they think that we should share the costs of health care through taxes, which is the way our medicare system is currently funded? If not, how should we pay for health care?

CHAPTER 4

Let's Get Healthier

In the remaining chapters we detail how to safeguard and improve medicare. Sprinkled throughout each chapter are clearly identified specific recommendations (in italics). You will find them also listed in appendix 1. We offer them as illustrations of how manageable the improvements to our medicare really are. They can serve as summaries that might prove useful in your conversations and correspondence with federal and provincial politicians.

This chapter is grounded in our conviction that governments have a role to play in preventing health problems and promoting good health outcomes. Libertarians and ultra-conservatives will probably not agree. When in 2011 the Danish government introduced a hefty tax on all foods that contained more than 2.3% saturated fat, some North American media disputed the right of any government to pass such legislation and questioned the wisdom of doing so; most of their objections were grounded in ideology and not insight. (Earlier this same government had put taxes on sugary junk foods [2010] and foods containing trans fats [2004].) We will not address the political and philosophical argument here other than to say that we also think that individuals bear responsibility for their health and should engage in sound practices that promote health and prevent illness. However, we are also convinced that there is room for proper government intervention, including campaigns to influence citizen choices. At the same time, we want to remain true to the principles of the *Canada Health Act*, meaning that every Canadian entering through a caregiver's door is entitled to receive care regardless of how they have lived their life up to that point.

The good news is that on the whole Canadians are getting healthier, and this positive trend is decades old already. The not-so-good news is that our health is improving more slowly than that of the citizens of some other countries. The second point can be illustrated by the following four studies.

Life expectancy is improving every year in almost every country, but Canada can do better. One study looked at potential years of life lost (PYLL). Although the study was complex, the result is easy to understand. Researchers selected a reasonable life expectancy age and then counted the years between actual death and life expectancy age as potential years of life lost. This study took 70 years as life expectancy age and then compared the ages at which people actually died in Canada, Australia, New Zealand, Sweden, Switzerland, the United Kingdom, and the United States. Over the decade 1994–2004, PYLL in Canada declined from 4,236 per 100,000 citizens to 3,365, an improvement of 2.3% per year. Over the same period this figure declined 2.7% per year in Australia and 3.5% per year in Switzerland. If we were to look only at Canada's statistics we would think we're doing fine. When you compare our results with those of some other nations, however, it is obvious we have room to improve.

PYLL is not the only tool used to make international health comparisons. In 2004 (the year of the Athens Olympics) the Conference Board of Canada published a report in which it considered a large number of health status factors and health outcomes. The study ranked countries as gold, silver, and bronze performers. On the basis of its criteria, it ranked Switzerland first, with a gold medal count of 37. Canada was ranked in the middle of the pack, coming in 13th place with a weighted count of 27 medals. We ranked 5th in health status, a shared 15th on non-medical factors, and a shared 20th on health outcomes (using PYLL measures and disease-specific mortality rates).

Another study looked at how eight major disease factors, individually and combined, affected PYLL70 performance (PYLL performance with 70 years used as the life expectancy age) in 26 developed countries. Canada's performance did not rank even third best when any of the eight disease factors were considered, nor in the overall PYLL rate. Canada's PYLL rate in this study was 3,365; Iceland's rate was 2,681, Sweden's was 2,929, and Switzerland's was 2,952. Overall, we ranked 8th out of 26 countries, and many other countries also performed much better than we did in disease-specific categories.

A study comparing Canadian provinces and territories using a similar method of analysis concluded that Ontario had the lowest PYLL, followed by British Columbia and Alberta. What should give us pause is the realization that if all provinces and territories achieved the PYLL rate of Ontario, there would be 778 fewer deaths in Canada each year per 100,000 population. (This study used a life expectancy of 75 years.)

These studies demonstrate that improvements in the health of Canada's population are possible. The trend to date has been for continuous improvements in life expectancy. However, if we are to catch up with other countries, more needs to be done. We need to determine what kind of interventions will yield the most improved health.

Thus far our analysis has focused on statistics concerning the average Canadian, but measures of health status (life expectancy and PYLL) are not evenly distributed. When we focus on gender, occupation, income, and location, we soon discover significant variations within our total population. For instance, aboriginal people suffer ill health more than other Canadians; life expectancies for First Nation and Inuit people are five to fourteen years shorter than for other Canadians. (Interestingly, new immigrants tend to arrive healthier than the average Canadian, but they lose that advantage over time.)

Another study compared the health issues of urban Canadians with incomes in the lowest third with the health issues of those with incomes in the highest third. The researchers looked at thirteen categories (e.g., injuries to children, birth weight, asthma in children, mental health, diabetes), and in each case poorer Canadians had more health issues. For example, more than twice as many poor Canadians suffered from chronic obstructive pulmonary disease (lung troubles) than rich Canadians did. Many other surveys have shown that poorer people have a lower life expectancy and suffer more from a variety of diseases. Other research seems to indicate that the health issues among poorer people have actually increased over the last decade. The data from all of these studies seem to argue for increased attention to the prevention of ill health among poorer people. Not only would pressure on health care budgets be lessened, but the life enjoyment of poorer people would increase.

This issue has been recognized before, at least implicitly. For instance, buried deep in the 2004 first ministers' statement on the future of health care was this recognition and commitment: "All governments recognize that public health efforts on health promotion, disease and injury prevention are critical to achieving better health outcomes for Canadians and contributing to the long-term sustainability of medicare by reducing pressure on the health care system ... governments commit to accelerate work on a pan-Canadian public health strategy. For the first time, governments will set goals and targets for improving the health status of Canadians through a collaborative process with experts. The Strategy will include efforts to address common risk factors, such as physical inactivity, and integrated disease strategies."

Efforts were initially made to implement the strategy. The Canadian Public Health Association, guided by a working group of the federal, provincial, and territorial governments, produced a discussion paper meant to "assist senior decision makers and other interested Canadians to contribute in an informed way to the development of Pan-Canadian public health goals." Using the paper, consultations were held throughout Canada. However, the final result, a 2005 document entitled "Health Goals for Canada" and inappropriately subtitled "A Federal, Provincial and Territorial *Commitment* to Canadians" [emphasis added], was disappointing. It contained "goals" but no targets. (Goals are nice, but targets pin down expectations.) It contained plenty of broad statements, such as "every person receives the support and information they [sic] need to make healthy choices."

The effort then went to sleep. The 2009 Senate Subcommittee on Population Health tried to awaken the sleeper by recommending in its report that "the Health Goals for Canada agreed upon in 2005 be revived and guide the development, implementation and monitoring of the pan-Canadian population health policy." But nothing much happened after that.

Similarly, every province has produced a set of health goals, but none has had a continuing impact on the health of Canadians. These goals generally lack specific, measurable targets accompanied by an accountability mechanism to guide the actions of stakeholders: wording such as "here are the specifics" and "here is how we shall measure success" is missing. It is with all this in mind that we offer our first policy initiative:

> *A pan-Canadian set of goals and targets for improving the health status of **all** Canadians should be developed by governments. Each province should then publish its own goals and targets, consistent with the national goals and targets. Regional health authorities and other*

organizations should also consider developing goals and targets consistent with the national goals and targets.

Health and Ill Health

However critical one might be about the genuine impact of government reports and actions on Canadian health, it cannot be denied that governments have been concerned. Back in 1974 the then Canadian minister of national health and welfare, Marc Lalonde, released a report entitled "A New Perspective on the Health of Canadians," which addressed four "health fields": human biology, environment, lifestyle, and health care organization. Eleven of the seventy-six pages in the report explicitly addressed the role of the federal government in improving the health of Canadians. Although the public health community hailed the report as a first in that it also addressed issues beyond immediate medical care, it ended up having little impact on policy. As is the case with many such reports, it was strong on analysis and weak on specific stimuli for action.

Others have built on Lalonde's notion that the health system is about more than care for immediate illnesses. Many researchers have since addressed wider issues that affect health, such as physical and social environments, genetic endowment, and individual responsibility. In past decades, genetic endowment was deemed to play a critical role in health. However, more recent studies suggest that this facet may not be as critical as once thought. More attention is now focused on the role of the physical environment, with one commentator using the term "environmental health justice." For instance, while on the face of it we all have access to a wide range of healthy foods, the actual choices are mediated through family and other social circumstances, in which incomes, habits, and awareness (or lack of it) play a large role. A sound health policy must recognize this interdependence of multiple factors. It is not easy to reverse lifestyle factors that may weaken health, as it may be necessary to break through social, economic, and physical constraints. For instance, a poor family living in a dense urban environment without a car may have (walking) access to only one supermarket whose marketing strategy is aimed at selling the most profitable goods, which most likely are the least nutritious. Choice is exceedingly limited in such circumstances.

Social and economic environments affect health as well. A sound pan-Canadian health strategy must therefore also address these elements and involve stakeholders beyond those directly involved in providing health care. If it is true that poverty has a negative impact on health (as we have already said), then poverty must be addressed, most urgently the plight of children living in poverty. How to do that is a complex matter, one often politically highly contested. Addressing poverty will take political will on the part of governments, and that will is constrained by voter attitudes and priorities. However, this remains true: addressing socio-economic and environmental factors is not only a way to improve health but also a way to make medicare more sustainable over the long term. Thanks to many researchers and writers, both popular and academic, the benefits of many measures have already been investigated and publicized. We have access to the right directions and the right roads to be taken. The question is: Can and will we start our engines? One first step is to highlight the various problems and then reiterate them regularly so we can track changes. Taking all this into account, we propose the following initiative:

Provinces and regional health authorities should publish regular reports on disparities in health outcomes.

So Let's Roll Up Our Sleeves

If medicare is to be sustained, reducing ill health is the place to start. Reducing ill health makes life better for everyone and it also lessens pressure on medicare budgets. However, many preventive measures that have proven health benefits may face initial social resistance. As always, the question of limits on government interference will be raised. We have already mentioned how Denmark introduced extra levies on foods high in trans and saturated fats as well as sugar, and these actions aroused the ideological ire of those who think that governments are far too intrusive.

We think there are areas where governments should intervene, but only if they have their priorities straight. For instance, should we focus on high-risk individuals (as some advocate), or on ill health issues in the broader population? With both of these priorities the causes of ill health will be addressed, but they require different strategies. For the first we target individual cases (how severe?); for the second we focus on the causes of incidence (how many?), on broad measures that affect the population at large. How does one decide which approach to take? To calculate the relative cost effectiveness of each approach we will need accurate information about which people are at high risk and the impact of interventions. Certain interventions may actually worsen health inequalities. The rich easily pick up on preventive health care messages and the poor might not. The experience with tobacco reduction interventions is a case in point: tobacco use among people in higher socio-economic groups dropped far more than among people in lower ones.

Tobacco

Overall there has been a remarkable decline in smoking in recent decades. In 2002, about one sixth of all deaths in Canada were linked to smoking, representing over half a million life years lost. In 1999 a quarter of Canadians smoked. However, by 2009 only 17.5% did. (It should be noted that the rate of decline has slowed in the last few years.) Tobacco consumption varies by education level: only 6% of university graduates smoked in 2009 whereas 19% of those who didn't complete high school were smokers.

The approach used in Canada to reduce (if not eliminate) tobacco use has not been limited to lifestyle issues, but rather it has also addressed social arrangements. The social context of smoking has been taken into account, and regulatory interventions have been adopted accordingly. Smoking has been increasingly banned in public places, and exposure to second-hand smoking has been restricted. Economic measures such as providing subsidies to quit smoking and increasing taxes on tobacco products have been shown to be successful. However, the tax measures in particular have been somewhat controversial, as they seem to have spawned cigarette smuggling and a market for contraband cigarettes. Moreover, cigarette taxes are regressive, in that the poor and the rich pay the same amount. There also may be a link between cigarette smoking and obesity: reducing the incidence of smoking may increase the incidence of obesity.

Revenues from court settlements with tobacco companies in the United States have been used to fund tobacco control programs, with California the shining example. By 2008 this state had reduced the percentage of its citizens who smoked to 13.3% (vs. 17% in Canada), it had got more people to quit, and it had slashed daily cigarette consumption as well as smoking-related mortality. Comprehensive control programs are still yielding benefits. We've made good progress in this domain, but there is more to do still.

Obesity

The growing prevalence of obesity is the contemporary *cause célèbre*. It has been described as an epidemic, a pandemic, a crisis, and a tsunami. Behind these dramatic words reside real issues: obesity increases the risks of mortality and premature death. The growing prevalence of obesity certainly will increase direct and indirect health care costs in the short run. Ironically, it may reduce net dollar costs, as the increased prevalence of obesity may actually decrease Canadian life expectancy.

It is tempting to declare obesity an individual lifestyle choice, given that it is produced by a combination of caloric intake and inadequate physical activity to use up the intake. However, food intake is heavily influenced by environmental factors, especially the social environment. Fast food outlets and supermarket designs have been identified as contributors to both overeating and unhealthy dietary choices. Cities are not designed for walking and biking. People watch sports rather than engage in them; incessant media coverage tempts them to remain on the sofa in front of the television. These are just some examples of the always-present pressures to eat poorly and forego exercise.

In 2003 two prominent Canadian health organizations convened a policy "round table" to identify actions to address obesity in Canada. The round table of course concluded that more research is needed (when it is ever not?), but it also recognized that the causes of obesity are complex and involve multiple factors. It proposed actions to be undertaken in schools, urban design and transport, and industry. The Canadian Heart Health Strategy and Action Plan (2008) outlined similar conclusions.

Alas, thus far Canadian policies to address obesity have focused on lifestyle interventions to encourage individuals to make better diet and exercise decisions. We clearly need a more balanced portfolio of strategies aimed not only at individuals, but also at organizations, communities, and institutions.

We may also need a series of economic incentives (taxes and subsidies). Although research results on the benefits of economic incentives are somewhat mixed, the case for a targeted tax on sugar-sweetened beverages is convincing. In addition to promoting health by lowering consumption of such beverages, the targeted tax would generate additional revenue that would help improve the long-term sustainability of public-sector health care. Introducing this tax will be an uphill battle. Stakeholders who produce and distribute these drinks will react with all the power they have as they will see consumption shrink. However, the example of increasing taxes on tobacco and restricting smoking opportunities should give us heart: these strategies worked. We therefore make the following policy recommendation:

> *The Canadian Health Services Research Foundation should be given the task to review the evidence on the use of tax incentives to promote public health objectives, including the case for a targeted tax on sugar-sweetened beverages.*

Strategies

Obesity and tobacco use are not the only public health issues. The field of public health is dynamic, and what may count as conventional wisdom today may become passé as new knowledge and new technologies emerge. Who knows what needs for legislative interventions may emerge within our lifetime?

Are there criteria by which to judge the legitimacy of legislative intervention, both in legal terms and in terms of public acceptance? We can think of at least one criterion that can be used to assess the legitimacy of interventions to improve the sustainability of medicare, namely value for money. Does an intervention produce enough positive benefits to warrant the costs of implementing it? Of course prevention is better than cure: it's better not to get sick at all. But not all interventions save costs in the end. The question is not whether we should prevent illness as much as possible: of course we should, individually and collectively. Rather, the question hinges on whether the state's investment in a specific intervention pays. By "pays" we mean more than sheer dollar outlay and returns. We also include, and by no means as by-products, health and social benefits.

Many writers have looked at this question. Over 2,500 health cost-effectiveness studies already exist, and many of those look at the cost effectiveness of specific preventive interventions. A catalogue of effective interventions is gradually emerging. For instance, vaccinating toddlers against *Haemophilis influenza* is effective, and so is colonoscopy screening for colorectal cancer in men 60–64 years of age. But screening all 65-year-olds for diabetes is a waste of money, and prostate-specific antigen (PSA) testing to detect prostate cancer early seems to be as well.

Cost-effective health studies from other countries can be helpful to Canadians. It wouldn't do to simply implement recommendations from abroad, as each country has a unique political and social culture and we may not achieve the same cost–benefit ratios with a given intervention. Furthermore, not every preventive intervention has been evaluated sufficiently. This is especially true for interventions to be used where significant social, physical, or economic disadvantage plays a prominent role, as we know from First Nations' experiences. There have also been fewer studies on interventions to address mental and behavioural conditions than on interventions for prominent diseases. A lot more investigative work is needed before a full array of promising interventions can be named. But if we are to be wise in our investments in this area, we'd better get moving on that investigative work.

Tips for you:
- Does your province (or territory) have a clear set of goals to improve health? Does it report on progress every year? (If so, does this report tell you whether it is doing better or worse than the rest of Canada?)
- If there is a provincial report, does it just provide provincial averages or does it also address concerns about the most needy in our society?

CHAPTER 5

Primary Care: The Foundation

Primary Health: The Foundation

Imagine a 50-year-old man who has a heart condition and has diabetes as well. His prospects for living a fulfilling, long life are good ... provided he takes good care of himself. Taking good care of himself does not require regular acute care, lengthy stays in hospitals in the care of high-priced physician specialists and well-trained nurses. He can continue to engage in productive work, play golf, go on holidays, make love, and volunteer. However, to take care of himself he does need a support system. The first line of support is found at his home, where his partner watches him and encourages him to take his meds and exercise, supervises his diet, and challenges him if he slips from the desired practices. The second line of defence is (or could be) his personal physician, a nutritionist, a nurse practitioner, and perhaps a social worker or psychologist to give him advice and encouragement when his biology indicates that his ways of living need to be changed. Notice that he requires not just a physician but rather a team of knowledgeable folks, who keep abreast of developments in the treatment of chronic conditions like his. In a perfect world all these health care providers are in the same office complex, and they all know his condition and needs. Ideally he will only need one appointment (from time to time) to see any of these people when he requires their help. He won't have to travel from one address to another, and he won't have to repeat the same information to people who have only their own specialty in mind. He will have a team of health care providers who have a joint focus on him. In between appointments they keep in touch via telephone and email.

That's the foundation, one advocated by many students of the health care system and beginning to be put into operation. But let us turn our minds away from that foundation and toward the still-overwhelming reality. What comes to your mind when you think of Canadians' health care? The media most often seem to focus on hospitals, and when they discuss our health care system they usually show a picture of one of our high-tech citadels. But most Canadians actually experience their health care in a local physician's office, not in a hospital. In 2007–08 about 22 million Canadians visited a physician, while in that same year hospitals discharged just over 2.5 million, slightly more than 10% of the number who saw a physician. For most Canadians a physician is the major link between them and our health care system.

What we propose in this chapter is the development of a system of primary care. It consists of a team of family doctors and other health care providers. A good primary care system can make a big difference to the health of Canadians and will cost less than our current health care systems. Quality primary care will ensure the proper use of the downstream parts of our health care system (diagnostics, specialists) and help control costs.

What is primary care? One observer defined it as "the means by which two goals of the health services system – optimization of health and equity in distributing resources – are balanced. It is the basic level of care provided equally to everyone. It addresses the most common problems in the community by providing preventive, curative, and rehabilitative services to maximize health and well-being. It integrates care when more than one health problem exists, and deals with the context in which illness exists and influences people's responses to the health problems. It is care that organizes and rationalizes the deployment of all resources, basic as well as specialized, directed at promoting, maintaining and improving health" (Starfield 1992).

In Canada a high-quality primary care system is more goal than reality at the moment, although efforts are being made. Starfield's description of primary care makes the important point that good primary care is the foundation for the functioning of the whole health care system. No wonder that in this chapter we advocate that resources be put to work to enhance and strengthen it. This spending will produce payoffs that will help keep medicare sustainable.

.Numerous studies have produced these consistent patterns:

1   Spending on primary care pays off in positive public health outcomes (some studies have even pointed to lower mortality rates).
2   Quality primary care services and preventive services should work in tandem.
3   With respect to health, primary care services can help to soften the impact of income inequality.
4   The availability of more primary care doctors will lessen the total cost of health services.

As we have said already, Canada's primary health care system isn't perfect yet. About 15% of all Canadians do not have a family doctor, and not all family practices provide the best primary care. One consequence is that hospital emergency departments are often full of anxious, sometimes bored, and often frustrated people: physicians, nurses, support staff, and patients all. The *Canada Health Act* ensures that finances are no barrier to access, a critical achievement and a good first step taken some 60 years ago. But access is about more than finances. It also means having health services available when they are needed.

A key reason to move away from single-physician family doctor offices is the fact that disease patterns and treatments have changed since the *Medical Care Act* was proclaimed in 1966 and the *Canada Health Act* in 1984. Fifty years ago acute care was the norm (in the acute care pattern, an individual gets sick, receives treatment, and, one hopes, gets better). Physicians worked in a fee-for-service system, in which they were rewarded for the specific treatment they provided. Today, the prevailing pattern is no longer that of acute care. The treatment of infectious diseases used to consume a lot of health care resources, but these diseases have been largely brought under control with preventive measures (inoculations, for instance).

In their practices today, physicians are far more concerned with monitoring and controlling chronic illnesses. These are the predominant causes of death, and their prevalence is increasing. In 1998–99 almost 13% of Canadians had hypertension whereas just under 20% of us did in 2006–07. In 2003 6.4% of Canadians suffered from diabetes; in 2006–07 that figure had increased to 8%. Given a Canadian population of 34 million, this means that in four years roughly 60,000 more Canadians had become diabetic.

Here is the impact of chronic diseases on health care. In 2007 the Ontario Chronic Disease Prevention Alliance in tandem with the Ontario Public Health Association produced a report with some startling information. The report looked at three groups of seniors: those aged 65–75 years, those aged 74–84 years, and those over 85 years. For all groups the following patterns were virtually identical.

- Each 1,000 seniors in each group made roughly 4,000 health care visits if they had no reported health conditions. That works out to a visit every three months on average.
- Each 1,000 seniors in each group made roughly 6,000 visits if they reported having one condition. (One visit every two months.)
- Each 1,000 seniors in each group made many more visits if they reported having two conditions (the youngest group roughly 7,600, the middle group about 9,600, and the oldest group just over 6,000).
- For three or more reported conditions, the youngest seniors made just under 14,000 visits, the middle ones about 11,500 visits, and the senior seniors 14,000 visits. These figures translate to an average of one or more visits to a physician each month by each senior in each group. Picture an 85-year-old having to do this, and think of the logistics, the anxiety each visit would produce, the time and energy each visit would take, and the resulting fatigue.

Here are some estimates of the direct costs associated with selected chronic diseases in all ages (year 2005 dollars; "direct" means a specific draw on health care budgets): $4.4 billion for cancers, $4.9 billion for musculo-skeletal conditions, $7.6 billion for cardiovascular diseases, $4.2 billion for diabetes, $10.4 billion for mental illness, and $3.8 billion for respiratory diseases. The total costs are over $35 billion. (As a wit once observed, a billion here and a billion there, and soon we're talking real money.) These figures highlight the significant costs of mental illness, which are twice as much as those for all cancers combined.

These direct costs are dwarfed by the indirect costs, which amount to an estimated $77 billion, more than twice the direct costs. This difference reflects the nature of chronic disease – some level of disability is an inherent part of the condition. Beyond personal discomfort (pain, reduced mobility), chronic disease exacts a monetary price through lost productivity and premature mortality. For example, people with complications of diabetes are more likely to be outside the labour force, and in total enjoy 28% less income than people without diabetes.

Here is what one commentator observed: "The reality of our time is that we are living longer, much longer, than previous generations. Yet, we are living longer not in perfect health, but with an array of chronic diseases such as diabetes, asthma, heart disease, arthritis, and others. Managing those diseases well is a major challenge facing aging Canadians. Helping us manage these chronic diseases is the major challenge facing the Canadian health system" (Decter 2007). To put this quote in a reassuring perspective, Canadians on the whole are healthier than they were in earlier generations, and many seniors are basically healthy, with only some of them suffering from one or more chronic diseases.

Chronic Disease Management

Chronic care demands a somewhat different approach than acute care. Acute care takes the form of diagnosis and a time-limited treatment that produces a cure. (For example, a broken leg gets set and is "casted" for healing in about six weeks.) Chronic care is about long-term symptom management, which requires ongoing care grounded in a trust relationship. Chronic care often requires different skills offered by a group of health care professionals. It also requires that patients realize that these professionals are not offering a cure but rather support to help them live as well as possible with the disease.

Unfortunately, coordination of the efforts of various health care professionals is often lacking. In 2007 30% of Canadians reported that their regular doctor's practice never or rarely coordinated care with other doctors. However, the tide seems to be turning. In many parts of Canada primary health care services are adopting innovative new models; even there is still a long way to go, this is a promising development.

System Reorientation

We badly need a transformation of the entire health system to service the needs of patients with one or more chronic illnesses. The emphasis should be on self-management. Descriptions of the health care system often start with a discussion of the services available rather than the needs (and responsibilities) of patients and their caregivers. Genuine person-centred care is still far from common. Figure 5.1 illustrates a way of visualizing a health care system that has the patient at its centre.

This model puts individual patients at the centre of his or her care package. It respects not only a patient's biology but also a patient's behaviour, culture, and values. Most people are healthy enough even if they have one or more chronic conditions, and they want to continue living productive lives. All support services are to be in the form of resources for living rather than barriers to living. In chapter 3 we defined our goal for the health system: *The right person enables the right care in the right setting, on time, every time.* The critical word is *enables.* A person with one or more chronic conditions can become his or her own expert, with the support of the health system. Skills for self-management can be taught (including the skills needed to access information on the internet confidently), and people so taught lead better lives. The research is unmistakable.

However, teaching self-management requires a systematic collaborative approach. The skills, interests, or resources to develop patient skills will not be available in every family practice. Family practices should be able to draw on a wide range

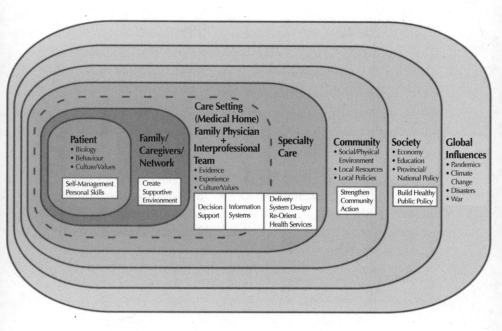

Figure 5.1: The patient at the centre of the health system

of resources, which will all need to be far more easily accessible than they are now. Evidence from existing programs is clear about the broad conditions that dramatically improve outcomes for chronic disease management:

- various types of physicians working together;
- involvement of such health care providers as nurses, dieticians, social workers, and pharmacists; and
- a program of encouragement for patients to change their behaviour through education and self-help skills training.

There are plenty of studies that document the benefits of this type of integrated care, in terms of both actual health and patient satisfaction. Lacking still are studies that document the impact on the cost of care. We expect that such studies will demonstrate substantial overall health care savings, for instance in reducing the number of physician visits by seniors with one or more chronic conditions.

Wagner's Chronic Care Model

We are not talking about an untried approach. Over the last twenty years, Seattle-based physician Ed Wagner has developed a comprehensive and multi-faceted approach to chronic illnesses. The model has since been implemented and evaluated in a number of places. At the heart of it is a "productive interaction" between "an informed, activated patient" and a "prepared, proactive practice *team* [italics added]" (Wagner et al. 2001). That team encompasses more than just physicians. Patient support is also provided by the wider community (through resources, policies, and support for self-management) as well as by the health system (with proper delivery of care and adequate clinical information systems).

We must remember that patients with chronic diseases live with their condition 24/7, and their partners do as well. There will probably also be an impact on the extended family. The "right person" will often be a family member or friend. The role of such a caregiver is to create a supportive environment for the chronically ill patient; this might involve making the home safe for walking around and other activities (such as showering and eating), assisting the patient with managing medications, and monitoring the patient's health. The wider community can support home modifications and provide support and assistance for caregivers, such as respite care.

This model goes beyond providing better, more comprehensive care. With chronic diseases becoming more prevalent, the enabling and supporting roles in the health care system (as opposed to the roles that simply involve the provision of care) become more important in the long run. We will need a larger health care workforce to provide the necessary medical care, but many of the ongoing care needs of people with chronic illnesses can be met by people with a narrower skill set, such as health care aides. Higher priced professionals can thereby be freed up to see a larger number of patients.

We are not proposing that responsibilities and costs be simply off-loaded onto patients' partners, family members, and friends. Patient training is key to self-management, but productive support by a range of caregivers is also needed. That support needs to be immediately available, and with the help of monitoring systems and the internet it can be.

Telephone advisory services (also called tele-nursing) will be crucial in this regard. (The Canadian Radio-television and Telecommunications Commission [CRTC] has allocated the number 811 for these services, and it is already in use in Nova Scotia, British Columbia, and Quebec.) Trained nurses use their skills and sophisticated computer software programs to provide triage as well as advice and support at a distance to caregivers and patients. Many patients still prefer to talk to their own physician face to face, of course, but studies have already shown that tele-nursing advice is followed well enough. A benefit of tele-nursing is that it is available at times when physician offices are closed. We're only at the beginning of this most promising health care development.

Of course, not all health services can be provided at home. The skills and knowledge of a primary care team of professionals will remain a vital component of health care: these professionals monitor and manage, intervening when a chronic condition destabilizes or acute episodes occur. However, the model of single-doctor practices is no longer sensible for primary care. The skills of the physician need to be supplemented by those of other professionals: nurses and nurse practitioners, people skilled in mental health, physical therapists, dieticians, and others. Such a team considers patients' needs from many angles.

Multiple-care family practices involving more than one physician will be able to be open longer hours and on weekends and so will also be available for some acute services, thus lessening the pressures on more expensive health care resources such as hospital emergency departments. Moreover, more personnel from other professions are often available in such practices than in a one-doctor practice. It should be recognized that this model is not a magic wand that will solve many problems quickly and reduce costs dramatically overnight. Much planning is needed, and current health care practitioners need to step back from their daily routines, analyze their current ways of doing things, and develop and implement improvement strategies.

The Role of Information Systems

It will come as no surprise that computers will play important roles in these new strategies. Computers are powerful tools for both storing and sharing information. Information and communication technologies have the potential to transform health care experiences. But the disappointing truth is that health care seems to lag behind other industries in capitalizing on this potential. Perhaps health care is fundamentally different from other industries. Sometimes computer program are introduced by well-meaning zealots pushing their cases too hard and too quickly. However, the potential is there to enable health care professionals to do their work well. We point to three applications of these technologies that are already in operation.

Remote Monitoring

Tele-care and remote patient management supports citizens to remain independent in their own homes through monitoring technologies, either automated (through some form of sensing), or through patient self-management (e.g., monitoring of vital signs and interactive voice recognition). Health care personnel call patients when reported data cross predetermined thresholds and trigger action. An extensive range of remote monitoring technologies is already available, and "smart home" programs have been developed in a several countries for a number of chronic conditions, such as heart failure and stroke. Many studies have already demonstrated positive health outcomes of these technologies, and some have provided economic analyses that provide hope.

In introducing and developing these technologies we must keep in mind that remote monitoring is about user (patient) needs. The push to implement must not be a mere technological push, one that disregards, for instance, the needs and perceptions of seniors.

Electronic Health Records and Personal Health Records

Electronic health records seem to be the Holy Grail of health electronic initiatives, and they have been lauded as the possessor of miraculous powers. Advocates say they will make health care safer, cheaper, and more integrated. They will prevent records being lost, eliminate duplication and inefficient billing procedures, and prevent mistaken identities, idiosyncratic clinical decisions, and drug errors.

However, things are not all that rosy (yet). We must distinguish between electronic health records and personal health records:

- Electronic health records are created to serve health care professionals, and they are in their hands. They are a repository of patient information that may be shared among health care providers and may help them care for their patients.
- Personal health records belong to an individual. They often partly reflect data from an electronic health record, but they are accessible by and often in the (electronic) hands of a patient. (Adrian and his wife Johanna have had such a personal record on their computer for years. They have kept a record of their medical history, including operations and interventions, as well as current drug use. They make sure it's current with the latest information and share it with any doctors they may have to consult, who invariably are grateful and impressed.) Personal health records can help patients with chronic illness to manage their condition(s), and we want the keeping of such a record made as easy as possible.

Personal health records can have a positive impact on health care. They can be vital links supporting patient self-management. By having (always current) information in their hands, patients will be able to take an active role in the management of their conditions. New forms are constantly being developed. A good one should track and monitor the patient's adherence to their medication regimen, for such adherence is positively linked to a reduction in the overall costs of the health system. Personal health records are still in the early days of development, but the fact that electronic giants such as Microsoft's HealthVault are developing digital platforms is a promising sign for the future.

The Romanow report (2002) recommended the "establishment of personal electronic health records for each Canadian." Alberta Health Services explored the implications of these records more recently. Encouragingly, the spur to that effort was improving patient service. One goal was "access to a personal electronic health record for anyone with diabetes, which will include their personal care plan and allow them to monitor and track their condition." Alberta Health Services intends to make personal health records available in multiple settings and with multiple users, employing new technology that is not dependent on existing institutional systems. So here is our next recommendation:

> *Health Canada should make available a personal health record platform for all Canadians; all provinces should work with Health Canada to facilitate populating the personal health record with provincially held data.*

Organizational Structures and Financial Incentives

We are convinced that the development of a sophisticated primary health care system is inevitable, given the pressures to keep medicare financially and economically viable. The road to such a system will be an uphill one, for a number of reasons.

We have already stressed that for Tommy Douglas' Saskatchewan the major concern was the catastrophic effects of serious illness (hospitalization) on a family's financial well-being. Physicians insisted that they remain autonomous and not become civil servants, and thus fee for service remained the primary remuneration structure of autonomous, single-physician primary care practices when medicare was introduced. With the evolution of primary care toward multi-disciplinary practice, a new financial incentive structure is needed.

Health care remuneration is a touchy subject. Many physicians will jealously guard their autonomy and their long-held key and leading role in health care. They will feel that it is essential that they own their practice and receive remuneration through the fee-for-service model. However, alternative forms of practice are already in place, in Canada and elsewhere. For instance, in university hospitals and private corporations, physicians are usually paid an annual salary that is not dependent on the number of patients they see or the number of services they perform. Although alternatives like these are in place at present, we have consistently made the case in this book that new delivery structures, accompanied by new forms of remuneration, are required as we shift the emphasis of the system from one designed to treat acute illness to one where chronic ailments demand a growing share of health care resources.

A single-physician practice is easy to run. It takes two people: the physician and his or her administrative assistant (who also serves as the receptionist). In contrast, a primary care clinic probably houses various types of physicians as well as therapists, nutritionists, nurse practitioners, other nurses, home care specialists, and support staff. With workers with a variety of skills functioning at a variety of income levels, institutional management problems can loom large. In a single-physician practice one person makes decisions, whereas in a multi-disciplinary clinic decisions are made by a team. To operate effectively, the team needs the utmost in cooperation, collaboration, and shared decision making, as well as a clearly understood authority structure with which all team members agree. Determining how power will be shared and exercised is of key importance. The challenges are considerable.

Nevertheless, the benefits of large multi-disciplinary teams are great; they can provide a "one-stop shop" so patients see the person with the right skills for their needs. In some cases this just means relocating existing providers so they work from the same home base. When professionals rub shoulders on a daily basis, communication and coordination are facilitated. The process of creating multi-disciplinary teams could start with developing closer links between physicians and home nurses.

We recommend the following policy:

Provinces should consider integration of home care and other community services with new (transformed) multi-disciplinary primary care practices.

Financial incentives can facilitate or inhibit good practice. There are three basic types of remuneration for physicians:

- set fee for specific service rendered;
- salary; and
- fee per patient.

The fee-for-service model is particularly inappropriate for primary care dominated by chronic diseases. It rewards discrete episodes of care rather than a long-term caring relationship. Moreover, it stands in the way of using, for instance, nurse practitioners for health care that will not necessarily require a licensed physician. Some studies already suggest that paying physicians for long-term specific patient care (the so-called capitation system) has positive effects on care. Forms of blended payment are being developed: fee-for-service payments could accommodate care provided after hours and abnormal care, fee-per-patient payments would reward physicians for the size of the practice, and a set salary would provide physicians with basic financial security. Achieving a blended payment structure that will be widely accepted will not be easy, and thus we recommend the following:

Provinces should review the structure of their payment arrangements for family physicians to ensure that they incorporate the right set of incentives for care of patients with chronic illnesses, including incentives that encourage physicians to support self-management, facilitate community-level interventions, and ensure the optimal division of labour.

Summary: An Integration Model

The initial and most frequent relationship between a patient and the health care system occurs in primary care. Primary care is the gate to other services, including home care, diagnostic services, specialist services, and acute services (e.g., hospitals). Effective relationships among all of those are a must. Integrated services are needed, with multiple disciplines working together. Many Canadian provinces are already moving in that direction with the development of regional health authorities, which typically incorporate hospitals and community services such as home care. A number of provinces have established regional groupings of primary care practices, a positive step toward integration of services.

However, organizational integration, with physicians working alongside professionals from an array of other health care fields, has not yet become a sufficiently large trend in Canada. The current emphasis on acute care and the resistance to change in health care structures stand in the way of organizational integration. Perhaps governments need to stimulate development through financial levers, which specify desired outcomes and how they are to be purchased; the UK government has already gone this route. Financial levers may include the possibility that an integrated primary care structure has (holds) its own budget. We will discuss this further in subsequent chapters, especially chapter 11. For now we recommend the following:

Provinces should review their primary care funding arrangements to ensure that funding streams are adequate to allow collaborative team practice.

Tips for you:
- Check the health stories in your newspaper over a one- or two-week period. How many are about hospital or research advances? When you see a story about primary care, write to the paper commending its editors and encouraging more stories about this important area.
- Can your family physician get access to your lab results online? If so, check with your regional health authority about their plans for you to get the same access.

CHAPTER 6

Pharmacare: The Time Is Right

We have already argued that greater efficiency will guarantee the survival of medicare. When economists talk about efficiency, they mean more than producing something at the lowest possible cost. Their concept of efficiency includes social efficiency, which involves the reaching of desirable ends. For instance, it is not socially efficient for people to frequent hospitals, which provide expensive care, simply because they don't have access to the right services in the community (which are much cheaper for governments and more beneficial for patients). Hospital care is simply not the best health care for certain conditions.

With social efficiency in mind, we recommend that we expand medicare to include pharmacare. In this chapter we'll make the economic case for this expansion. Pharmacare will help us to control the amount of money now spent on pharmaceuticals, and will have a positive impact on health.

The creators of medicare did not make explicit provision for access to drugs, except where these are provided within hospital walls. Today, provinces have variable programs for drug coverage, but most of them are highly inadequate for needs that did not exist before. Patients with significant chronic conditions often require expensive drugs and may face financial hardship in accessing them. Foxy patients sometimes manage to get themselves into hospitals simply to gain access to the drugs they need. More tragically, seniors under financial pressure get tempted not to take their drugs; if they don't comply with their treatment their health suffers and ultimately acute care costs rise for their province.

Let's look at the feasibility of making pharmacare a component of medicare. In 2009 pharmaceutical expenditures constituted about one sixth of total health care spending. Drug costs were paid for by insurance companies (via employment or individual premiums), directly by Canadians, or via provincial subsidies.

The pharmaceutical share of total health care spending has grown markedly in recent years, from 9.5% in 1985 to 16.4% in 2009. The public proportion of drug spending has grown in that time from 29% to 38%, and private spending has also increased because of higher overall spending. It is disconcerting to discover that, because of costs, in 2010 about 10% of Canadians did not have their prescriptions filled or skipped doses. When they neglect to take their medications, more serious acute conditions requiring expensive (acute) treatments are likely to follow. This trend was already evident at the time of the 2002 Kirby report, prompting the authors to observe that "no Canadian should suffer undue financial hardship as a result of having to pay health care bills" and to assert that "it is essential that this principle be applied to prescription drug expenses" (Kirby 2002, 125).

In 2009, the average Canadian spent $893 on pharmaceuticals. Spending ranged from $714 in British Columbia to $1,057 in Nova Scotia. What accounts for such a substantial difference within the borders of one country? Age and gender variations in provincial populations explain part of the difference, but the major factor is per prescription volumes and different patterns of pharmaceutical prescribing. The cost is different if you get a prescription for a year's supply versus a three-month supply of a medication. Quebec spends about 13% more than could be expected given its population, and it also has a far above average number of prescriptions for smaller prescription volumes. The differences indicate the potential for cost savings in some provinces if a more equitable pharmaceutical system is developed for the whole of Canada.

A sound pharmaceutical policy covers three main elements:

- safety and efficacy;
- equitable access; and
- responsible prescribing.

Canada is doing well in the first area. We seldom hear of catastrophes resulting from the use of unsafe drugs or from sudden shortages. However, Canada has some way to go on the other two elements, particularly equitable access. Canada has no national drug provision policy, and provincial ones fall far short of creating an equitable system for all. A number of authors have concluded that:

(a) we spend far more on drugs than we need to, and the costs are rising faster than elsewhere;
(b) access to this health need is not equitable right now; and
(c) subsidies to the pharmaceutical industry do not produce sufficient benefits for all.

Table 6.1 clearly shows that we spend more than almost all other countries on patented and generic drugs.

Europeans (apart from the Swiss) spent much less than we did to get patented and generic drugs. Americans paid more than we did for patented drugs, but this finding should not make us happy. Clearly we pay far too much for drugs.

So what needs to be done?

For reasons of both equitable access and cost, Canada clearly needs a national pharmacare program. It is an urgent matter,

Table 6.1 *Average relative unit prices for pharmaceuticals, compared with prices in Canada, adjusted using market exchange rates*

	Canada	France	Italy	Germany
Patented drugs, 2010	1.00	0.90	0.87	1.20
Generic drugs, using pharmacy acquisition cost, 2008	1.00	0.73	0.70	0.62

	Sweden	Switzerland	United Kingdom	United States
Patented drugs, 2010	0.98	1.03	0.86	1.91
Generic drugs, using pharmacy acquisition cost, 2008	0.42	1.12	0.54	0.57

as many chronic diseases are kept in check with the help of drugs. Such a program should also address issues of efficient purchasing and should include sound policies for determining which drugs are to be included. Several studies have already determined that substantial costs saving could be gained with a sound national policy that avoids costly provincial duplication.

Gagnon (2010) is one of the commentators who have offered concrete suggestions on how a pharmacare program could be developed. He highlights, for instance, the virtues of more efficient purchasing and a quality assessment program for determining which pharmaceuticals to include in the program. Other researchers have suggested that the existence of a single national list of included drugs would be an immediate and substantial cost saver. Moreover, the use of generic drugs could be greatly enhanced with timely and appropriate encouragement to pre-scribers and patients.

None of these and other measures will be easy to implement, even if the overall potential savings to Canada's health care system are clear. Gagnon has this to say.

> Let's not be naïve: establishing a national, universal drug plan providing first-dollar coverage is not a simple matter. Government funding, even when lower than comparable private spending, is often extremely difficult to justify publicly. A national pharmacare program will have to find a balanced approach to ensure coherence across the country while respecting provincial health jurisdictions. But these are not insurmountable obstacles. Quite the con-trary. A clear policy backed by real political will would allow all Canadians to have equal and universal access to the best treatments available, while generating substan-tial savings over the current plans. The analysis in [my] report shows that the only hindrance to establishing a fair, effective drug insurance program is political apathy, not economic or cost restraints.

Political apathy is not the only barrier. There is sure to be strong opposition from vested interests (notably pharmaceutical and insurance companies), and the media will be full of ideological arguments. Many will object to the fact that a national pharma-care program will increase the public sector's role in medicare, but as a number of authors have shown, the national savings would be substantial.

To come back to the concept of social efficiency, equitable access to drugs will help ensure the optimal treatment for chronic illnesses, given that most of these treatments depend on pharmaceuticals. Proper intake of drugs will lessen sudden demands for (expensive) acute care and hospital visits. The following discussion makes the case more narrowly for cost savings.

In 2009, Canada spent about $25.4 billion on prescribed medications, of which $11.4 billion came out of the public pot and $9.4 billion from insurance companies; $4.6 billion had to be coughed up by individual Canadians. Modifying Gagnon's ideas a bit, let's say we make prescription medications an insured service under medicare. We establish a national pharmaceuticals list as well as national purchasing (item A). Moreover, we abolish those insurance company premiums and replace them with provincial prescription premiums to the tune of approximately the same $9.4 billion (item B), with some provision for co-payments (item C). The immediate financial impact of items B and C together would be cost neutral (premiums would be paid to the provinces rather than to insurance companies, and individuals would still pay a portion of their drug costs). Item A has the potential to save considerable money, lessening overall health care costs.

The researched information leads us to suggest that:

Prescription drugs should be an insured service under medicare. Federal, provincial, and territorial leaders should immediately commission an independent study to determine the most practical way of introducing prescription pharmaceuticals as an insured service under medicare.

A tip for you:
Write to your member of Parliament and your provincial political representative and ask them what their policy is about updating medicare to cover pharmaceuticals outside hospitals.

CHAPTER 7

Innovations in Health Care: Who Benefits?

We live in an age of unprecedented innovation in many areas of our lives. Health care is no exception. There is a steady flow of new drugs, new tools, new equipment, and new procedures. The first answer to the question in this chapter's title is that untold millions have already benefited from innovations in health care.

Adrian and his wife Johanna have personally experienced the blessings of innovations. Adrian had to have his appendix removed about one month after he landed in Canada in 1954. His belly was cut open, and he had to stay in the hospital for one full week then spend another week recovering at home. He thus lost two weeks of work. The large scar on his belly is a permanent reminder of his surgery. Someone requiring an appendectomy today would probably have it done laparoscopically, be home the day after the procedure, and be back at work in a few days. The only restriction would be to avoid heavy lifting for awhile. A laparoscopic procedure was used to remove part of the meniscus from Adrian's right knee in 1992. It was done in a hospital in the morning, he was sent home in late afternoon with instructions to start serious exercise the next morning, and in less than a week he discarded his crutches. At first the three small incisions where the "tube" had gone in were visible, but you couldn't find them today. New procedures like this one produce shorter hospital stays, lessen the chance of infections, and dramatically improve patients' experience during recovery.

In 1988 Johanna visited her family physician for a regular checkup. He got worried when he could not see her optic nerve and sent her straight to a local hospital, where she immediately received a spinal tap. After a few days in the hospital and many tests she was given a diagnosis of pseudotumour cerebri, a process that acts like, but is not, a brain tumour. To combat the symptoms (too much fluid retention), she was given heavy diuretics (which, by the way, damaged her stomach sufficiently after a while that she will have to take medicine to suppress upset stomach symptoms for the rest of her life). Unfortunately MRIS were not available in 1988. In the 1990s she underwent an MRI test, and it was discovered that she had a real brain tumour, which was very small and fortunately not cancerous. A specialist monitored her every six months, and she had an MRI test every 12 months; in 2004 the specialist decided to remove the tumour as it was growing slowly but steadily. The operation was a success. It took 8 hours on a Wednesday. On Friday morning the surgeon told Johanna she could go home, and she resumed her regular routines two days later. How can one not marvel at the blessings of technology?

Laparoscopic surgical techniques and MRI machines are two splendid advancements among many. Of course, some innovations do not turn out so well. There have been reports recently in the media about the breast implant scandal in France and about newly developed artificial hips that break inside some patients in Canada. On the whole, however, we can only marvel at what clever brains, skillful hands, and compassionate hearts are achieving for us.

In the rest of this chapter we will take a closer look at how these innovations come to be and whence they originate. We'll discover that all is not well, and that they can be used more efficiently, taking into account social efficiency, or, in other words, the health benefits to patients.

New Technologies and Procedures

Outside the health sector the introduction of a new technology is almost always a cost-saving measure. In contrast, in the health sector, cost savings cannot be the major emphasis: new technologies are most often designed to enhance quality, for instance in reducing the side effects of an existing treatment, reducing the invasiveness of a procedure, or tackling previously untreatable conditions. In tandem with rising incomes, public health interventions, and other factors, innovations in health care have most certainly contributed to the decline in mortality rates. However, they have come at a cost, perhaps in the range of between one quarter and one half of the annual increase in per capita health spending over the last 40 years, not only in Canada but in all developed countries. As we have already argued, aging, demographics, and tax base problems cannot account for the steady increase in health care costs beyond the rate of inflation. Instead, we must look at the impact of both new technologies and new drugs on spending.

Some new technologies produce only small benefits. Some are quite expensive. Others are cost effective with some patient groups and not with others. How do we decide which ones to implement? Policy-makers are turning their attention more and more to strategies that will ensure that new technologies are worth their costs. They are creating policies that press for economic evaluations and assessments about whether new technologies should be included in health policy coverage or other funding models.

At the national level, the Canadian Agency for Drugs and Technologies in Health (CADTH) conducts health technology assessments. Other organizations also conduct such assessments, such as provincial governments, regional health authorities, and hospitals. However, as Romanow (2002, 83) observed, there is a lack of information sharing and plenty of assessment duplication.

Two basic questions are at the heart of health technology assessments.

1 What is the nature of the evidence about the cost effectiveness of the new technology?
2 How much will it cost to implement the technology?

Determining cost effectiveness involves weighing inputs and outputs, outlays and benefits. However, the valuation of benefits is an inexact science. There are frequently tensions between societal values, as expressed through political decisions, and benefits as reported in academic studies. Studies funded by corporations are particularly vulnerable to subtle bias. For instance, the groups of patients selected for research studies may differ from the patients typically seen in regular practice. Unfortunately, most new technologies do not get evaluated systematically in normal practice settings.

Even so, let us assume that the information provided by evaluation studies is valid. This question then arises: Should cost effectiveness information determine coverage decisions? The brief answer is no. Use of a technology may be ethically warranted, or even indicated, even if it cannot be shown to be cost effective. Here is a real-life example. Adrian served as a member of the ethics committee of a major hospital for a time. One of the cases under scrutiny concerned the use of a drug that would cost the hospital well over $100,000, which would prolong the life of a patient for no more than six months. However, the patient's medical crisis had arisen suddenly, and she was the mother of three young children. Use of the drug would give her time to prepare her children for her death. The committee recommended that the drug be provided to the patient and the hospital agreed, even though the hospital was aware that using the $100,000 elsewhere could benefit many more "ordinary" patients. The patient received the drug.

We advocate the judicious use of new technologies. We must make sure they are evaluated properly, not only in terms of safety and efficacy but also in terms of cost. We need to approve the implementation of new technologies with our eyes wide open about what the new drugs or machines will do and what we will have to pay for them. Will they be worth it, or do we want our precious health care dollars spent on something low tech, such as more home care?

Academic Health Science Centres

Academic health science centres (university hospitals) have important roles to play in the development of innovations. In principle, the research that is pursued at these institutions will lead to innovations that are then tested and implemented on a large scale. The process involves five steps: conducting research in the basis sciences; developing a new technology, procedure or drug; trying it out; sharing the information gathered during testing; and teaching clinicians to use it.

The temptation is for institutions to restrict activities to only those that can occur within their walls (i.e., the first three steps) The fourth step (publishing the results of testing) is left up to the individual researchers, and the fifth step requires initiative on the part of clinicians to acquaint themselves with the innovation and implement it, wherever they may be in practice.

Why are the last two steps left up to individuals? Many observers have commented that prestige and status matter a lot in universities. In academic health science centres, prestige is showered on researchers who produce advances in basic biomedical science, and these individuals often are richly rewarded in the form of personal income and future grants. Unfortunately, research down the line in the process has less status. It takes a lot of hard and patient slogging, most of it behind the scenes, to get a (perhaps brilliant) development into full clinical practice. If the five steps are not seen to dovetail as part of an integrated process, the time between the initial research finding and wide implementation of the resulting innovation can sometimes stretch to as much as ten years.

We are suggesting that universities should become much more active outside their walls in disseminating the new technologies that they have invented or developed, in teaching and training clinicians to use them, and in evaluating the impact of new technologies not just on those patients they see in their own locations, which are often well-equipped with state-of-the art tools, but also in less endowed, smaller, and more remote locations. We therefore recommend that:

Academic health science centres should document and publicize to their students how their research actually leads to improvements in efficiency in the delivery of care.

A tip for you:
Does the faculty of medicine at your nearest university produce an annual report on research? Get hold of a copy or search the university's website to check out what they are doing to disseminate their findings to local family physicians.

CHAPTER 8

Those Seniors Once More

We began chapter 5 with a dream for primary care. In it we pictured the ongoing care for a middle-aged man with chronic conditions. If we can realize that dream by developing primary care clinics for everyone, then life for all seniors will become easier and more pleasant, at least with respect to the health care they will need. However, more needs to be done for seniors. This chapter tackles the gap between the care received by seniors still living at home with or without some kind of support and that received by seniors in total-care nursing homes. To fill that gap we advocate expansion of home care and the rapid development of assisted living facilities, which provide a mid-level residential care service with a range of supports for senior residents.

Current Status

Aging is about becoming frailer (although one hopes to also become wiser). Seniors normally do not grow old alone. Their immediate supports, namely their wives, husbands, partners, and friends, tend to be close to their age. Sometimes our care needs increase gradually as we age, but often they increase in fits and starts because of acute events (like a stroke). Our potential supports may have their own care needs and may be able to offer only limited support. Almost all seniors may come to rely on some degree of help from strangers.

The current seniors' service system is poorly designed and riddled with discontinuities. The care provided in hospitals and by services outside the hospital does not mesh, and neither do home care and residential care. There are also serious gaps between "health" and "social" care. Individual seniors may not get appropriate service, and the service they do get may be far more costly than is necessary. For instance, seniors may remain in hospital for want of better care in a more suitable and less expensive location. There is no coherent national approach to long-term care. One observer has said we have a mosaic of inequalities within our nation and even within each province. Sometimes terms have different meanings in different provinces (e.g., nursing home, assisted living facility, hostel, lodge), and there is no national data collecting mechanism. Statistics Canada produces a report on residential care facilities, but it does not include information about which residents need, and receive, what kind of care. Confusion and inequality result in resources being wasted as well. Seniors deserve better.

Here are a number of statistics from 2008–09 that we have gleaned from the information available. In that period there were about 2,200 seniors' residences in Canada, which cared for more than 200,000 residents, 3% more than in the previous year. (The rate of increase in the number of seniors living in seniors' residences is probably even higher now.)

- Most of these senior residents lived in large facilities of 100 beds or more (a third of the total facilities).
- Only about 9% of seniors lived in facilities with fewer than fifty beds.
- 45% of the facilities were for profit, accounting for about 44% of the beds.
- Half of the residents were 85 years of age and over; 20% were between 80 and 84.
- 70% of the residents were women.

The distribution of beds varies from province to province. Prince Edward Island has the highest number of beds per population of citizens over age 65, namely 14.2 per 1,000; Alberta has the lowest (5.1 – but it has a younger population) and Quebec the second lowest (5.2).

In addition, on any given day about 5,200 acute care hospital beds are occupied by people who no longer need acute care but for whom residential care or home care is not available. Patients provided with what is often referred to as an alternate level of care tend to be older than other hospital patients (median age 80 compared to 63), and about 4% of them stay more than 100 days. A goodly proportion of these beds are taken up by people with dementia.

43% of patients who had been classified as receiving an alternate level of care were discharged into a long-term care facility, 27% were discharged into a home with some support, and 12% died. 17% of patients who had received an alternate level of care while in hospital were readmitted within 30 days (compared with 12% of other patients). Ontario, the only province to provide these data, reported that 27% of senior patients who had been discharged from the hospital had an emergency department visit within 30 days of discharge (versus 22% of other patients).

The gap really begins to show in the next set of statistics. The majority of seniors do not live in residential care settings. Only 14% of people over age 85 do. Of people over age 90, 60% of all males and 53% of all females live in a single dwelling. (Of course, the definition of home may change. Empty nesters move into smaller dwellings, often either apartments or seniors' complexes.) These figures make a strong case for home care, both formal and informal, as the dominant form of support. In 2003 about 563,000 people received some form of support in their homes, with almost three quarters of them receiving care from formal sources. These may be government-subsidized health care or homemaker services, or care purchased from private agencies or provided by volunteers. Informal care provided by family and friends often supplements formal care, with 15% of the 563,000 receiving care from both formal and informal sources. About two thirds of home care recipients were assisted with housework, with just under one third receiving nursing care.

Of course, some seniors need to be looked after exclusively by professionals. Seniors in a total care facility are likely to be people with Alzheimer disease, people with urinary incontinence, people over 85, and single people without a support system of family or friends. For others, however, home care at its best is able to respond to a broad range of health, social, and personal needs: housework, nursing and other health care, personal care, meal preparation and (or) delivery, shopping, recreation, and respite. Needs may be short term or ongoing.

There is much need for home care. Although the number of people receiving government-subsidized home care increased between 1994 and 2003, the proportion of people over age 65 receiving such care fell almost 4%, most notably because of a drop in support for housework.

Home Care: What Needs to Be Done?

Seniors' care covers a continuum from the simple to the complicated, from shopping and housework, through wound care and monitoring, to dressing and feeding. However, there is not a matching continuum of care provision. Different facilities offer different packages and elements of care, but the greatest discontinuity is found in the fact that once a patient is discharged from the hospital, the *Canada Health Act* becomes inoperative for the provision of pharmaceuticals and health care beyond hospital and doctor visits. That gap jeopardizes continuing care for those with limited means. It is clear that the services to meet seniors' needs must be expanded, and patient care should be at the centre of our attention.

There can be no doubt that any reform should begin with establishing a secure and stable home care program. From a home care funding perspective, home care may prevent or postpone hospital admission for people with chronic illnesses, thus reducing the need for a much more costly form of care. The need for better home care has been recognized for many years. In 2002, for instance, Romanow called home care "the next essential service."

Home care has four major components, which can be illustrated with these questions: Who should receive it? What should they receive? Who pays? What is the impact of care?

Assessment and Access

Who should receive home care? As with any government service, there has to be an equitable system to determine eligibility. Unfortunately, at present there is no common provincial system for assessment and classification. A number of provinces are beginning to standardize a system covering assessment for a range of settings, including home care and residential aged care (which includes both nursing home and assisted living residences). The system uses a standard set of questions, avoids duplication in assessments for different settings, and is aimed at ensuring consistency in the way the needs of a particular senior are being assessed. The system (called interRAI) is also used in a number of other countries.

But there is more to assessment than collecting the answers to a standard set of questions. It also involves clinical judgments by a professional about the strength or fragility of informal networks of support; usually such judgments are made by nurses trained in seniors' needs. Even so, Ontario encountered difficulties as it implemented the interRAI assessment system. The following lessons have been learned.

- A proper program of standardized assessment is likely to uncover unmet needs and inadequacies in the current systems. Is the existing system open to changes in management as well as the provision of appropriate resources? Often it is not, given that institutions are used to taking their time to respond to real needs.
- A proper computerized information system is essential.
- Clinicians, managers, and policy-makers must receive ongoing education in the use of assessment and informational instruments.
- Feedback is critical, and data must inform decision making at all levels of the health care system.
- Although data may be used in a variety of ways, the emphasis must be on clinical applications regarding daily care provision.

Assessment, however well done, is only a first step. If it is to produce positive results, the personal care and health care services shown to be needed by the assessments must be available. As we have already said, at present there are too many discontinuities, even wide gaps.

Self-managed Care

Over the last decade, in Canada and elsewhere, enhancing choice has been a characteristic of seniors' care policy. It is no longer true that the inability to live safely at home inevitably means a move to a nursing home. More types of residential care

are available now in nursing homes and assisted living residences. Within residential aged care facilities, residents are gain-
ing more autonomy and choice. Enhanced home support options
are being developed that help seniors to avoid moving into a residential aged care facility altogether. Personal budgets, which
are already part of the care provided to adults under age 65 who
have disabilities, are being considered for seniors. This service
involves giving an individual the responsibility for a personal
budget, set after client assessment, with which they may purchase
the services they need. Providing personal budgets for seniors
has become standard practice in several European countries, and
a number of Canadian provinces are experimenting with them.
These self-managed care programs are potentially much more
tailored to the specific needs of seniors and their caregivers and
allow a high degree of flexibility in and responsiveness of the care
when conditions change.

Personal care budgets, like all forms of self-management,
must satisfy a number of prerequisites.

- A standardized assessment approach is needed to
  ensure equity in resource allocation. Equity demands
  that specific cost allocations in a particular client's
  personal budget be aligned with those for similar
  clients in traditional home care or residential programs. Negotiations with the client or the client's
  principal caregiver must take place regarding the
  resources provided.
- The budget needs to be adequate to meet the needs
  of those who want to self-manage their care. They
  should neither be favoured over clients in standard
  seniors' care arrangements nor be subject to tighter
  resources.
- The services included in the personal care budget
  must indeed be available.

- Accountability is required, as these are public funds.

Self-managed care is not without its critics. Some point out the risk of abuse. Clients and needs not formerly known to the system suddenly appear as the system is implemented, and volunteers suddenly want to get paid. However, some empirical evidence suggests that this effect may be small and need not impair the approach. Moreover, proper assessment procedures and caps on expenditures per client can ensure the efficient use of resources. All of this is sufficient for us to suggest that:

Provinces should incorporate self-managed care as an integral part of their home care systems.

Co-payments

Seniors' hospital care doesn't demand personal contributions (except perhaps for parking). By contrast, personal contributions for senior care are common outside of hospitals. This is not unreasonable, as these contributions may include housekeeping and shopping expenses, which healthy people normally have to cover out of their own pockets. Then again, residential aged care facilities do pay for food, light, and power, in addition to the health care provided by nurses and other personal care workers. So, who should pay for what? It is reasonable to expect seniors to pay for the equivalent of normal household expenses. However, for health care services, it should make no difference whether these are offered within hospitals, in other facilities, or at home. When these services are offered free in hospitals but not at home, longer stays in hospitals may be engineered, subtly or bluntly. Inequity results in higher health care public budgets. We therefore propose the following policy initiative:

Seniors' health care, whether provided in the home or in a residential aged care facility, should become an insured service under the Canada Health Act.

This initiative wouldn't completely solve the prospective financial tensions between personal expenses and health care expenses in seniors' facilities. As aging persons become more dependent, the dividing lines between the two types of expenses may become more blurred. Let's look at shopping as an example. People living independently spend their own time shopping and pay for their purchases out of their own pockets. But if a seniors' facility shops for its residents, it must pay workers to do it. Also, a residential care facility may offer services not available in an ordinary home (entertainment, libraries, and exercise programs for instance), and it may cost more to house a resident in the facility than it would cost if the individual were living on their own. The cost of preparing food also has to be considered. Perhaps some personal costs should be subsidized.

Subsidies (and differential co-payments) will also be required to ensure equity. At present provinces have different standards and different income thresholds for subsidies and co-payments. Provincial co-payment policies do not seem to take into account the fact that the cost of living may vary depending on where one lives. Low real estate values in certain areas may not be reflected in the price of living in a local seniors' care facility, presenting problems for homeowners in these areas who are compelled by their health and other care needs to sell their homes: they may receive far less for the sale of their home than owners in other parts of the country.

Impact

Home care works. Integrated systems of home care for seniors reduce use of institutions, shorten hospital stays for patient requiring an alternate level of care, and hence save money. No wonder the trend is away from institutional care and toward keeping seniors in their homes with various forms of support. This trend can be seen not only in Canada but also internationally. It doesn't matter much that different settings have different costs. All home care options cost governments less than institutional care. Both the Kirby and Romanow reports advocated home care; as we mentioned earlier, Romanow called it "the next essential service."

Ensuring Quality in Residential Care

When home care becomes impossible, residential care is a next stage for seniors. Residents in residential aged care facilities tend to be more frail and vulnerable than people at home. Many experience cognitive impairment, and a surveillance and regulatory system needs to be in place to protect their interests. However, as international records show, at present the provincial regulatory systems for aged care are flawed. Institutions often end up focusing on facility rituals; for instance, they may insist that documentation be completed correctly even if the care that is being provided is incorrect, or they may focus on writing rules, not on getting treatment problems fixed. Abuse can occur, and abuse scandals are periodically reported in the media. We clearly need to reform regulations.

Some provinces do not have any regulations at all. In those that do, the regulations call for a mix of inspection and rewards or incentives. Traditional inspection methods can now be supplemented by quantitative measures derived from assessment and reassessment processes. The aforementioned interRAI system incorporates specific quality measures across twelve clinically oriented domains. They're listed here, to indicate the breadth of assessment: accidents, behavioural and emotional patterns, clinical management, cognitive functioning, elimination and continence, infection control, nutrition and eating, physical functioning, psychotropic drug use, quality of life, sensory function and communication, and skin care.

The incidence and prevalence of any of these could be used as part of a regulatory framework, as a basis for inspection, in public reporting, or as part of an incentive payment system. (Home care should have a similar set of quality measures, and in some cases those are already available.)

The US Centers for Medicaid and Medicare Services operate a website called Nursing Home Compare that rates nursing homes on the basis of health inspection results. It appears that nursing home managers, not consumers, are the main users of the website: they use it to check how their facility is being rated and try to fix identified problem areas. US nursing homes often compete for favourable referrals from physicians, and a high rating helps. US commentators have pointed out that the quality of nursing homes increased overall a few years after public reporting was implemented. We suggest that:

Provinces should explore the possibility of publicly reporting the quality of nursing home care.

Public reporting alone is not enough. Other initiatives will be required, such as instituting a properly staffed long-term care ombudsman's office. Clinical features are not the only dimensions of seniors' care, and quality measurements must also capture these other features. Especially in assisted living facilities, such domains as preservation of independence and autonomy are critical. Some researchers have begun work to address quality standards in these institutions. As with primary care, a culture of mere "doing" that is examined only from the staff's perspective needs to be replaced by a culture in which the focus is on seniors' care. In many institutions this will require an extensive culture change.

Expanding Residential Care Options

Until some years ago, there was a gap between home care and care for people who require nursing homes. Nursing homes are designed for the most dependent elderly, and they provide 24/7 coverage by registered nurses. The residents of nursing homes are likely to have complex clinical needs, and hence the facilities have an atmosphere that is more like a clinic than a home. There clearly is a need for seniors' residences that provide intermediate services. Assisted living facilities have begun to fill this gap, providing additional options for seniors and providing a continuity of services for seniors whose needs may increase as they age.

For instance, some seniors may initially only need some supervision and reminders and perhaps minimal assistance with respect to bathing, dressing, and personal hygiene. Gradually they may grow to need more assistance with these activities and perhaps also with eating; at some stage they may require assistance with all activities of daily living, including personal hygiene, incontinence care, moving, and feeding.

Nursing care may initially only be a matter of coordination with a health care provider (nurse or doctor), but it may grow into more intense consultation, assessment, and scheduled direct care (e.g., wound care), and may ultimately involve 24/7 monitoring and reacting to incidents.

With respect to orientation and behaviours, residents may initially only require reminders with occasional interventions, and then they may need regular reminders, prompts, and direction along with interventions in response to occasional disruptive of intrusive behaviours; and they might finally require a structured behavioural program.

Nursing homes serve the needs of seniors who need constant supervision and care in three dimensions: personal care, nursing care, and behavioural supervision. However, some seniors do not need care in all three of these dimensions. Assisted living facilities can provide a more flexible staffing arrangement with a mix of staff (not all need to be registered nurses) and thus accommodate a mix of residents. Good ones may even be able to accept people almost at nursing home levels of dependency but whose nursing care needs are less demanding.

The notion of assisted living is still developing in Canada. In many parts of Canada assisted living facilities are not yet available, forcing seniors into nursing homes prematurely and at great cost. Therefore we recommend the following policy initiative:

> *Provinces should encourage and facilitate development*
> *of a broader range of accommodation options for*
> *seniors, including an intermediate residential care*
> *option, assisted living.*

Funding Residential Care Facilities

There are enormous variations in the funding arrangements for residential aged care services across Canada, and even within provinces. Here's a case in point. Until recently each regional health authority in Alberta developed its own funding formula for these services. In some cases each facility negotiated its own capital funding arrangement, with confusion reigning regarding care and accommodation costs. When a pan-province Alberta Health Services board was established, it set out to introduce consistent and equitable funding of care needs across the province, using interRAI to assess the needs of individual residents. It discovered that payments for the same type of resident ranged from $100 per day to well over $400 across the 180 nursing homes funded by Alberta Health Services. There is every reason to believe that similar differences in funding exist in other provinces.

There may be a way to equalize funding (and perhaps save funds overall) by promoting activity-based funding in every province, which would entail developing a formula so that the funding that goes to a residential care facility is based only on each resident's needs. That would ensure equitable funding, as all residential care facilities would get the same amount for looking after residents who require the same level of care. Of course, there may be some differences across provinces, for instance in how capital costs are funded, how "hotel" costs and care costs are distinguished, and what income thresholds are established.

We recommend the following policy initiative:

Provinces should aim for activity-based funding for residential care.

Summary: The Need for Reform in Seniors' Care

In chapter 3 we articulated the following goal for Canadian medicare: *The right person enables the right care in the right setting, on time, every time.* Addressing seniors' need in the right setting is critical if we are to sustain our medicare.

Doomsayers usually simply extend the current utilization and service mix into the future and tell us we can't afford medicare forever because our population is aging. In chapters 2 and 3 we countered this attack. In this chapter we outlined how changing seniors' health strategies can help us control costs and provide far better care for an aging population. We think that expansion of services and improvements in efficiency (cost and social) can proceed side by side.

Tips for you:
- Does your province have an intermediate level of residential care similar to assisted living? What are the province's plans for providing more residential care in light of the aging of the population? How many additional beds are needed per year? How many of these will be assisted living beds? What will be the proportion of nursing home to assisted living beds in 2020?
- Are there long waiting lists for access to home care? What are the province's plans in this regard?

CHAPTER 9

Hospitals: Quality, Access, and Efficiency

Hospitals are complex institutions staffed by highly educated and trained caregivers. They also have a long tradition of strong hierarchies. In this chapter we will touch on only some of their complexities. In the end, hospital care will be improved only if there is what we will call a just and trusting culture within each hospital. As in other areas of health care, we remain convinced that genuine progress will not be made until health care workers are given room to tackle their problems themselves. Only then will administrative prodding toward efficiency (including social efficiency) and provincial government policies (e.g., forms of funding) become effective in achieving savings and providing just care. We are convinced that major savings are possible. This chapter is meant to be a prodding chapter.

Who looks forward to going into a hospital as a patient? Neither of us do, although we are thankful that hospitals are there should we need one. Although it provides lodging and food and may even look like a hotel, a hospital is not a place of enjoyment. (However, Adrian recently heard a story of a man in his 90s who was recently widowed and who has physical handicaps that severely restrict his social life. As soon as this man experiences discomfort he wants someone to dial 911 to get him an ambulance to rush him to the nearest hospital. He loves being in that hospital, where nurses know him and where he gets fussed over all day and night. It beats being in a small apartment on his own all day.)

Many of us have a sense of awe about hospitals, even if we don't want to stay in one. Hospitals can be thought of as the cathedrals of the 21st century. In medieval times cathedrals were centres of inspiration and truth in which miracles could take place. They were also centres of power and wealth, and around them revolved the life of a city. Indeed, miracles do occur in hospitals, although they are of a scientific kind. So when you stand underneath a vaulted roof in a hospital atrium, you may be filled with cathedral-type awe.

But that awe is being undermined these days. Regularly the media report that in this or that Canadian hospital patients pick up infections that seem resistant to almost all antibiotics. Then newspapers pounce on the inadequacy and insufficiency of the cleaning staff and on the nurses and doctors (who they claim are overworked and negligent and don't even wash their hands every time they should). They might also blame all of us for being too reliant on antibiotics. Even taking into account the penchant of newspapers to seek out the bad and exaggerate the damage, the elements of truth in these stories undermine Canadians' trust in hospitals. Trust is an essential component of healing, and no one wants to enter hospital doors afraid that the hospital itself may cause further ill health.

In an emergency, we want hospital care. At their best, hospitals offer rapid diagnosis, a highly trained staff, and treatments that save lives. They offer surgical care, address causes of pain, and help improve daily life. But should hospitals be the centres of health care, as cathedrals were the centres of soul care? Should patients and health care services revolve around hospitals? We don't think so, as we have already said and implied. Anyway, this model is under challenge, with policy reforms in many countries focusing more on primary and chronic care and less on acute care.

Let us repeat our goal for a health system: *The right person enables the right care in the right setting, on time, every time.* As we have already observed a number of times, the *on time* and *every time* components of this goal are not always available, and neither is *right care* in the *right setting.* Newspapers regularly report long waiting times and other hospital deficiencies, including concerns about patient safety.

Hospital Quality: The Safe Care, the Right Care, Every Time

In 2003 the Canadian Patient Safety Institute was established, in response to alarming reports about hospital patient safety. Concerns about patient safety had especially and dramatically come to the fore in both the United States and the United Kingdom. Quality is broader than safety; it includes acceptability, accessibility, appropriateness, effectiveness, and efficiency (and the latter includes social efficiency). For instance, acceptability highlights the tension that sometimes exists between what clinicians advocate and what patients value. We'll discuss this further later.

What do we know about hospital safety in Canada? One major study showed that an adverse event occurred in roughly 7.5% (one in fourteen) of all hospital admissions, with higher rates in teaching hospitals (10.3%). In about 20% of those cases death was the result. Adverse events tend to result in extra days of care, which of course piles financial woes on top of moral ones. ("Do no harm" is one of the bedrock ethical aspects of health care.) Reviewers concluded that in about one third of those events, the adverse event could have been prevented. Canadian rates are in line with those found in other countries that compile similar performance reviews.

Safety is only one of the issues that must be addressed. Various countries have discovered that key quality improvements require a change in hospital culture most of all. A two-fold culture change is required:

- a just and trusting culture must be established; and
- a culture of efficient teamwork must be created.

Let's look at these two factors in more detail.

A Just and Trusting Culture: Owning Up to the Wrong and Intervening

Fifty years ago almost everyone was convinced that the health care system rarely made mistakes; if something did go wrong, the blame was usually put on some errant individual. Views have changed since then. We now accept that systemic mistakes happen in the health care system as in other systems. Health care providers are willing to learn from mistakes so they do not happen again. Individual faults used to be the starting point for analyzing what went wrong. Now we think about mistakes in terms of concepts like "web of causation" and we talk about the fact that there are multiple contributing factors, many of which are organizational and systemic. Creating a just and trusting culture is an important step in the creation of a culture of safety. Even if individuals know they are at fault, a just and trusting culture will encourage them to report their error, and this opens the door to allow everyone to learn from mistakes.

Freedom to report is one key element of a just and trusting culture; freedom to intervene is another. Health care organizations tend to be strongly hierarchical, and it isn't easy for someone down the ladder to raise safety issues involving people higher up. Moreover, media tend to sensationalize quality issues and then pounce on the individuals they select as responsible. Politicians sometimes do this too, as they are used to finding fault elsewhere.

As some researchers have reported, achieving measurable change has not been easy. At the conceptual level it isn't difficult to describe the contours of a just and trusting culture.

However, it is trickier to describe it more precisely, and a common definition and agreed-upon measurements are required. Without an agreed-upon definition, it is hard to settle on consistent measurements. A number of definitions have been offered, but different researchers seem to focus on different elements. Definitions and measurements cannot become the norms for action if these butt heads with the organizational culture. If measuring is step one, step two involves changing the culture. This involves multiple interventions, including broad safety and management education programs.

Many interventions have been undertaken to improve patient safety in health care facilities across Canada and abroad, but few have been rigorously evaluated, at least as revealed by published studies. In spite of some efforts to create a common vocabulary for incident reporting, notably by the World Health Organization, there is little consistency in the way incidents are reported or analyzed. As a result, it is difficult for one institution to learn from the experiences of another.

Given all that, we recommend that:

The Canadian Patient Safety Institute should develop guidelines for incident reporting systems and mechanisms to share lessons from incident reviews across Canada.

As we said, good detection depends on the existence of a just and trusting culture that encourages the identification and reporting of adverse events and near misses. The introduction of periodic and regular incident reporting has been shown to increase detection. The development of a method for extracting a set of "patient safety indicators" from routine administrative data (diagnoses and procedures) has also contributed. Both these reporting systems provide ways of summarizing and

classifying reported adverse events in each individual hospital. Such valuable information should also be shared, within
and between provinces.

Efficient Teamwork

A second element in culture transformation is the building of
more effective health care teams. Entrenched hierarchies tend
to impede teamwork.

It's hard to think of a hospital care intervention that does not
involve transitions of care from one professional to another.
When Adrian served as spiritual caregiver in a hospital he often
observed nurse shift changes, a time when tired nurses leave and
fresh nurses arrive. Just before the end of their shift, nurses were
busy updating charts to be used by the nurses in the next shift.
At other times he observed patients being transferred from one
institution to another. During either one of these transitions
information may be lost or misconstrued. Test results may not
travel across settings or may be misplaced in poor handovers
between shifts and during inter-hospital transfers. Adverse
effects are most often attributed to communication lapses, but
these may also be symptoms of intra-organizational conflicts.

Patients expect efficient teamwork. Effective teamwork depends
on trust and on knowing what role each member plays and what
skills she or he has. Effective teams easily combine the contributions of motivated individual team members. They encourage
everyone in the team to participate in assessing team contributions. Effective hospital teams do exist, but unfortunately on the
whole published studies do not (yet?) provide clear direction
on how to create and maintain high-functioning teams.

Hospital clinical teams also have a key role to play in improving efficiency in processes of care (see also below). Moreover,
they provide a forum for reducing variability in clinical processes. Continued study toward a specific quality improvement

is necessary until a process has become standardized and the measured aim has been achieved. Teams can be powerful mechanisms for sharing and learning, especially if learning is based on evidence. Standardization can present challenges to some clinicians who highly value their autonomy, but autonomy should be valued insofar as, and only insofar as, it contributes to better outcomes.

Effectiveness and the Challenge of Variation

Quality and safety in hospital health care depend on reporting what may have gone wrong, especially when a death is the result. However, as more than one observer has pointed out, the next emphasis should be on implementing practices that improve quality across the board, not just with respect to safety issues. Implementing sound practices that are based on evidence is the key. There is already plenty of evidence pointing to many sound practices, but implementation often lags behind the release of such evidence. To ensure that a quality improvement measure is actually implemented, the evidence supporting it must be easily accessible at the bedside and there must be follow-up.

Over the last few years attention has begun to focus on one aspect of evidence-based practice, namely variation in medical care. Most of the research in this area has been conducted in the United States. An article in the *New Yorker* (June 2009) examined the contrasting experience of two Texas towns with vastly different hospital admission and utilization rates. We have known for a long time that variation in hospital utilization (both admission rates and length of stay) also exists in Canada, between and within provinces, but this knowledge has not led to the widespread adoption of improved practices. Canada needs more solid research. For one thing, higher hospital utilization rates do not necessarily guarantee improved outcomes. Hence we recommend the following policy initiative:

The Canadian Institute for Health Information should be given the task and be funded to expand publication of data on variation in utilization rates across Canada.

Perhaps some hospitals are underused, some are overused, and some have it right. We need to find out which ones are in each group, and why. How can the first and second groups reach the level of the third? It will take a number of strategies to achieve the right level of utilization for each hospital, including informed patient choice with respect to ethical and legal standards that govern elective surgeries, drugs, tests and other procedures, and care at life's end. The science of health care delivery needs to be improved so that undisciplined growth in health care capacity and spending can be reined in. Part of that improvement must include greater participation by patients.

Promoting Choice

When evidence is inconclusive, clinicians can legitimately differ in their treatment recommendations. As some have suggested, the hand of the patient in the decision-making process should be strengthened in such situations. Different patients will have different valuations; some will lean to surgery and some to watchful waiting with an eye on changes in signs and symptoms. Their decision may differ from a surgeon's advice. One observer suggested the following ways to assist patients to make decisions (called patient decision aids by Stacey et al. 2011):

- Provide reliable information about the patient's health condition and the options with their associated benefits, harms, probabilities, and scientific uncertainties, preferably tailored to the probable outcomes given the patient's age and health status.

- Help patients clarify, either implicitly or explicitly, the value they place on the benefits, potential harms, and scientific uncertainties.

We would add another factor, namely ensuring that a patient's sense of hospital awe does not stand in the way of his or her full participation in decision making.

Those patient decision aids have already been shown to influence patient choices, resulting in lower rates of surgery and improved patient satisfaction, but they are not yet a common part of regular practice. Perhaps financial incentives and a new legal standard could encourage wider use of patient aids. Consent forms could include materials from patients' aids and could be tailored to the characteristics of individual patients.

Improving the Science of Hospital Care

We advocate a greater involvement of patients in decisions about their acute care treatment in hospitals. In many cases there is a zone of complexity, which lies between the absolute certainty of treatment being vital on one side of the spectrum and the clear indication of preference on the other. This zone of complexity is where patient input can be given greater prominence. However, it is also the zone about which we need to know more and then share more.

That will require a much more systematic approach to clinical practice and clinical innovation than is common today. Today clinical practice is often an outflow of the preferences and styles of particular practitioners in particular settings. What is needed is an increased standardization of approaches to care. Studies have already shown that standardized pathways reduce complications in hospitals and probably lengths of stay. Standardization requires in-house clinical leadership and teamwork.

Moreover, it should involve learning from other facilities, learning from a study of variations, and being well aware of local practice idiosyncrasies, which may or may not prove valuable.

In Canada such learning could be stimulated by the creation of provincial clinical networks, in which health professionals working in different types of care and different disciplines in different locations would be linked to share information and insights. There is no reason that teams in one province shouldn't link with similar teams in another. Such networks already exist in the United Kingdom and Australia. Such teams would have the expertise to develop standard pathways, practice approaches, and methods of comparing clinical performance. The strength of these links is that they are grounded in clinical practice. Hence we recommend that:

Provinces should create and fund clinical networks to provide leadership in sharing good practice to improve access to health care and the quality and sustainability of health care.

Such links easily have another benefit, namely that specific locations will become known for their success with standardized procedures and will perform a high volume of those procedures. Research is clear: volume reduces complications. Of course, caring for patients in hospitals some distance from their home will always involve trade-offs between clinical outcomes and such factors as increased travel for patient and visitors, not to speak of the local politics of removing specific services from some hospitals and locating them in one centralized hospital. Different patients will make different decisions. Changes will probably be gradual, with most patients initially preferring to be treated locally (or as close to home as possible). However, when it becomes known that outcomes in centralized treatment locations are superior, more and more patients will be willing to travel. The change will depend on having reliable information about outcomes.

Given the success of this pathway to superior service, clinical networks can also become the authorizing bodies for evidence-based standardized treatments, replacing the often-inconsistent multiple guidance sources now in place.

The *Canada Health Act* obliges provinces to cover "necessary" services, a vague and undefined concept (see chapter 1). Perhaps greater precision could be achieved if we added a qualifier such as "effective," provided that provinces would then not also implicitly add a resource qualifier, as in "effective given the resources." Two approaches could mitigate that risk:

- All provincial processes to assess effectiveness should be transparent and independent of government.
- A national body (such as the Canadian Agency for Drugs and Technologies in Health) could establish a register of technologies deemed ineffective, with provinces having to exclude those, thus establishing a national core of common covered services.

Both approaches could be pursued, and effectiveness as a criterion for coverage could stimulate effectiveness research in Canada. Hence we recommend the following policy initiative:

The comprehensiveness criterion in the Canada Health Act *should be amended to include an obligation on the part of provinces to cover effective services, with a requirement that effectiveness be determined in a transparent way.*

Access: Getting the Right Care, On Time

This is well known: a built bed becomes a filled bed. Additional supply (of beds and physicians) leads to additional use but not necessarily to improvements in health or patient satisfaction. In addition, more nursing home beds do not necessarily lead to fewer acute hospital beds, which seems counterintuitive. However, this supply effect is unmistakable in both rural and urban areas. The process is akin to new metropolitan expressways not alleviating traffic jams for very long.

Some provinces have far higher hospitalization rates than others. In 1995–96 these rates ranged from a high of more than 14,000 per 100,000 population in New Brunswick and Saskatchewan to a low of under 10,000 in Quebec and Ontario. By 2005–06 there had been an overall reduction of about 25%, but the comparative pattern remained virtually the same. Saskatchewan had dropped to around 12,000, New Brunswick was still second highest with well over 10,000, and Ontario had dropped to well below 8,000 per 100,000 population.

Decisions about the availability of hospital beds are complex, tough, and political. Decisions may not always be solely related to health, or even health care, and relations between local authorities and funders can become testy. What should govern decisions is a rigorous criterion for admissions and a monitoring of the appropriateness of admissions and length of stay, taking into account social factors. Expansion proposals should also be reviewed and compared with the possibilities of using existing hospitals or developing community-based alternatives, which are most cost effective. Hence we make the following policy recommendation:

Provinces should request clinical networks (when established) to review intra- and inter-provincial utilization rate differences. Networks should be invited to develop or update priority-setting criteria.

Canadians know that they have to wait too long for access to primary care, specialist care, emergency care, and elective care. Canadian waiting times are longer than those in many other countries. Even Canada's tracking of waiting times is patchy and inconsistent. There is no standardization of definitions between provinces and sometimes not even within provinces. Reporting is often focused only on five priority areas, which were originally mentioned in the 2004 accord: hip and knee replacement, cataract surgery, coronary artery bypass grafting, diagnostic imaging (MRI and CT), and radiation therapy. There is no evidence that these five areas are trustworthy indicators for the performance of the whole system, and we should exchange this five-sided emphasis for a more comprehensive approach.

For instance, a patient waiting for an elective procedure counts the days between the referral by his or her family physician and the time when the operation occurs. However, public reporting typically focuses on the days between a surgeon's decision that a procedure is warranted and the performance of the procedure. There is no magic bullet that will fix wait times. No single strategy, uniformly applied, will alleviate the problem. The causes and symptoms of waiting lists vary across Canada. Nevertheless, there are three common elements that must be examined to tackle the problem: measurements and target issues, demand and supply issues, and efficiency issues. Let's have a look at all three.

Measurement and Target Issues

Here are some of the factors that complicate the development of standard definitions.

- For elective procedures, the total wait from family physician to procedure should be included. Components of the wait, such as time before specialist consultation and time between specialist decision and hospital availability, should also be measured. Where is the largest waiting time? Moreover, is there a gap between the date a patient receives all necessary information and the date he or she decides to go ahead with the procedure? Should the calculations be based on census reports or actual patient experiences? It is likely that some patients included on long waiting lists will actually no longer belong on those.

We therefore suggest that:

Provinces should commit to adopting common definitions of waiting times for the full patient journey.

- Measurement goes beyond simple counting. A consistent priority-setting process needs to be in place to ensure that urgent cases are dealt with expeditiously.
- Measurement without targets is futile. Incentives with targets accompanied by rewards and sanctions have proven to be successful in shortening waiting lists. The United Kingdom has successfully used this approach to dramatically reduce waiting times. Quebec, in response to a Supreme Court decision, has introduced a guarantee, with patients having redress when targets are not achieved.

So, with respect to measurement, we recommend the following policy initiative:

Federal, provincial, and territorial leaders should agree to waiting time ranges for a broad range of services. Provinces should publish consistent data on their achievement of those targets at least quarterly; these data should be collated and published nationally by the Canadian Institute for Health Information at least annually.

Demand and Supply Issues

On the demand side we once more take a look at both the growth of the Canadian population and its steady aging. These factors are increasing demand. However, as we have already discussed, other factors mediate this growth. We think of the following:

- programs that aim at improving our health;
- programs that question the tendency to believe that all health issues need intervention; and
- programs that suggest alternative treatment options.

Future demand does not have to be an extension of current demand. Health care approaches and public perceptions can change. Changing the overall culture will be a lengthy process, but some immediate steps can help. Implementation of informed patient decision making is one such strategy. Improving management of chronic illnesses is another.

Demand and supply should be in balance. Demand, for instance, has to do with how many people arrive each hour in an emergency department and how many arrive in primary care each day; it is a measurement of flow. Supply may be expressed in terms of how many patients are treated in the same time periods.

A mere counting of supply spaces (family physicians or hospital beds, for instance) is inadequate. The emphasis should be on how these supply spaces perform. Capacity is one factor, but productivity is another important one.

Efficiency Issues

Unit costs of care (e.g., cost per patient, laboratory test, or physician visit) vary considerable across the health system, both within and between provinces. Some of this variation arises from waste in the system as a result of overly complex administration, some is operational waste, and some is social waste: the right care is not being provided in the right setting. Let's have a look at all three.

Administrative Waste The Canadian health system is not overly top heavy, certainly not in comparison with the health system in the United States. During the 1990s a wave of provincial reviews eliminated countless separate small health boards and thus overhead. Of course the trend toward regionalization does not guarantee the elimination of waste, and it is true that forecast savings are seldom actually realized. However, notwithstanding the criticisms of centralization that are always present, consolidating Alberta's nine health regions and three provincial boards has led to significant reductions in the number of senior administrators as well as to savings through economies of scale in purchasing and other functions.

Operational Waste Under the pressure of increasing costs over the past decade, techniques to improve workflows and processes to eliminate various forms of waste have been widely implemented. In the health care sector, it is fundamental that improvements be made in the flow of patients from referral to rehabilitation, in operating room procedures for both elective and emergency cases, and in the procedures leading up to, and away from, operations, such as intensive care. Although outside consultants are often called in to improve flow, key is the involvement of those in the workplace who will be affected by the changes.

Poor quality care can produce operational waste associated with longer stays, returns to the operating room, avoidable emergency room attendance at the end of life, and avoidable readmissions. Many observers suggest that efficiency and quality go together. One large study concluded that medication errors and falls were areas where the greatest efficiency gains are likely to be found. This conclusion challenged the value of the often-suggested restrictions on nursing care and other operational expenses.

Clinical Waste Clinical waste can be produced with services that provide few marginal health benefits over less costly alternatives. A US study singled out eight standard procedures, the overuse of which cost the system 1.9% of all health spending, a massive amount in dollars. Three of them are as follows:

- excessive use of antibiotics for viral upper respiratory infections;
- avoidable emergency department use; and
- inappropriate hysterectomies.

Others have used the term "marginal medicine" for the same phenomenon and have applied the term to the use of interventions without adequate evidence of net benefit, to the use of a particular intervention when other options are cheaper, and to the use of high-cost procedures that only produce incremental benefits.

As we have already mentioned, clinical waste also has to do with inappropriate care for patients requiring an alternate level of care. It is estimated that alternate care patients occupy about 5,200 acute care beds across Canada on any given day. Clinical waste occurs when patients are admitted with a condition that could have been prevented with adequate primary care and timely intervention, for instance with prior use of a vaccine. These (ambulatory care sensitive) cases accounted for one in eight hospital admissions in 2006–07. Rates of these sorts of admissions vary widely across Canada, a solid sign that it should be possible to reduce these admissions almost everywhere. Better chronic disease management (discussed in chapter 5) and investments in home care (chapter 8) would dramatically reduce these admission rates and the associated costs. Moreover, sometimes acute treatment can be provided at home. The outcomes of such "hospital at home" treatments have been shown not to differ from those with in-patient treatment and they are of course less expensive. Failure to use such programs is another form of waste.

Additional waste occurs with the overuse of laboratory tests and diagnostic imaging as well as excessive lengths of hospital stays. The use of experienced physiotherapists in orthopedic care reduces the need for visits to a surgeon, as does the use of specialist nurses in orthopedic clinics.

Using procedures with proven low clinical value is another form of clinical waste, such as performing a hysterectomy in cases of heavy menstrual bleeding, extracting wisdom teeth, conducting cosmetic procedures such as orthodontics, and performing tonsillectomies. Recognizing that there may be disagreement about these items, guidelines in the United Kingdom suggest that appropriate reductions in these and other items could yield a per capita savings of $15 (for 33 million Canadians, this translates to over half a billion dollars). The Good Stewardship Working Group in the United States came up with a list of the top five ways to improve the quality and cost effectiveness of internal medicine, family practice, and pediatrics, which would also yield massive savings.

Why are we harping about waste? Put it in the context of public debates about the cost of health care. Our view is that part of the way we will ensure medicare remains sustainable is to eliminate waste. In fact, we'll go further; we think it is immoral to cut services if waste abounds.

Incentives for Improving Efficiency

There is increased focus on the different methods of funding hospitals and other segments of the health care system. Past and current methods are coming under scrutiny as they are not providing the right incentives to managers to address contemporary problems such as the need to improve efficiency.

There is increasing interest in Canada and elsewhere in the technique of service-based funding (we prefer to call it activity-based funding) as a spur toward greater efficiency; it was recommended in the Kirby (2002) report. The idea is simple: hospitals and other sectors get paid on the basis of what they do (i.e., on the basis of their activity). They receive a specified amount for each care job.

Activity-based funding has two key elements:

- revenue is directly linked to the volume and acuity of patients treated; and
- payment per patient is independent of a specific hospital or other service.

Unfortunately, there isn't widespread agreement on its implementation. For instance, opinions differ on whether facility funding should be capped and what methods should be used to describe what the facility does (activity). On the positive side, in the United States activity-based funding for medicare patients in hospitals has been in place for almost 30 years and has proven its merits.

Activity-based funding has been shown to spur managers to make significant improvements in efficiency. However, it may be difficult to implement activity-based funding. Activity-based funding may affect hospital power structures, as hospital managers are likely to put pressure on physicians to reduce the number of services they order (e.g., lab tests and diagnostic imaging) and lengths of stay, in combination with implementing strategies to reduce the costs of services ordered. Not all hospital departments are equally efficient, and pushes for efficiency may cause some intra-facility conflicts.

Activity-based funding cannot be implemented overnight. Hospitals should be given time to prepare for it and should be supported with the required management infrastructure. On the positive side, activity-based funding may spur increased demand for hospital substitutes (such as home care). All this leads us to recommend the following policy initiative:

Provinces should commit to a phased introduction of activity-based funding to drive improvements in efficiency in the hospital sector and other sectors.

Canada's health care system is run provincially, with decentralization of funding policies within provinces. These conditions will likely cause substantial variations in costs per patient treated across Canada. Care must be taken to ensure that while each province develops its own activity-based funding approach, provincial variations are not incorporated into the design, except with good cause.

Hospitals are the most visible symbols of health care, but they are also the most expensive ones. Getting hospital and acute care right would be a welcome indication that health care is indeed sustainable, and of course in and of itself higher efficiency would produce considerable cost savings. This chapter has tried to document the fact that many efforts are being made to increase the efficiency (both cost and social) of hospital care but that no magic bullet has been found as yet (if ever there will be one) to suddenly improve quality, access, and sustainability. As must be clear by now, these three are linked. As should also be clear, progress will likely be incremental.

A tip for you:
How are hospital budgets determined in your province? Are they related to activity or based on politics and negotiations? Does the province publish the costs of treatments in different hospitals?

CHAPTER 10

Nurturing and Obtaining the Right Skills

Here is the heart of this chapter: health care professionals are bright, they have received many years of education and apprenticeship, and they naturally want to use their competence to the full.

Sometimes a health professional is called to be a lone Good Samaritan, for instance in caring for a sick fellow passenger in an airplane or caring at the roadside for someone hurt in a collision. But such individual care is rare these days. Contemporary health care involves professionals and support staff working together. Perhaps our health care goal (see chapter 3) needs to read: *The **right member of the health care team** enables the right care in the right setting, on time, every time.* This caveat should be kept in mind: family members and caregivers in the patient's social network are also part of any such team.

An appropriate team is central to good quality care, but it is not always available. Barriers to a balanced workforce can be found within the health care system, and they may not be immediately fixable. These barriers include the presence of individual and collective career choices, regulations currently in force, and levels of compensation. We must also consider barriers from without, such as the prevailing economic conditions. An example of the latter would be high unemployment in one part of the country and low unemployment in another, with positions going unfilled in the latter area.

The health care workforce challenge is often simplified to be merely an issue of one or another health care profession being short of bodies. This is not the place to start worrying. For one thing, such a focus inevitably leads to workforce planning mistakes. Here is how we think planning should proceed:

1 The proper starting point for planning is the identification of future health care needs.
2 We then consider actions that would respond to those needs.
3 Next, we imagine the kind of workers who would execute those actions.
4 Finally we estimate how many of those workers might be needed.

Workforce planning mistakes are inevitable if they are based on an unchallenged assumption that the existing division of labour in health care is an unchangeable norm. As we saw in the previous chapter, health care systems vary a great deal from region to region, and thus even today it is questionable whether there is an ideal division of labour. Furthermore, the evidence that supply leads to better health outcomes is highly debatable. The demand side of the health care workforce (What needs are to be met? What work is to be done? What skills are needed? How many people do we need?) should run parallel with the supply side (Who will occupy the various posts?). Let's have a closer look at both sides.

The Demand Side

Health care workers determine the very nature of health care. Given all the changes we have suggested earlier in this book, we should carefully reflect on their future roles. Professional health care is already changing and will need to evolve even more in the years ahead. In comparison with today, there should be (will be) more emphasis on supported self-management and an expansion in assisted living, as we have already argued at length. The shift from treating acute to chronic illness is another development. Existing skills are not likely to disappear, but they will receive a changed emphasis. Skill will not only be measured in terms of an individual's technical competence, but rather it will also encompass the ability to communicate, work in teams, see patients as persons in social contexts, and so on. The Royal College of Physicians and Surgeons of Canada believes that physicians must be competent in multiple roles: the central role is that of medical expert, but physicians must also be competent communicators, collaborators, health advocates, managers, scholars, and professionals. The roles each have a set of defined competencies, but they are interwoven. Similar lists of roles could easily be created for other health care professions.

Life magazine's Norman Rockwell and 1950s TV shows portrayed physicians as omniscient and omnipotent. Although these portrayals were factually wrong, they perhaps reflected public perceptions. The rapid expansion of diagnostic and therapeutic services since then has made the public understand far better that health care is a partnership, with many professionals making contributions. Functions that were carried out exclusively by physicians in the past are now part of the skill sets of many other professionals. For instance, two-year hospital-based training for registered nurses has been replaced with a four-year university-based preparation. In a number of provinces, licensed practical nurses now receive that two-year training.

For the moment, however, current task descriptions (reflected in regulatory bodies' legislation) do not reflect sufficiently the competencies that many health care professionals have gained in their academic preparation and subsequent experience and continuing education. That disconnect between education and job descriptions causes enormous professional frustration, which often comes to express itself in sideways battles. For instance, in some health care contexts the disconnect has led to contests between unions and management for more: more status, more power, and more money. We think that contacts between employers and employees should be guided to facilitate mutually acceptable developments toward cost-effective, high-quality, and accessible health care that requires everyone to offer the utmost of their skills and dedication.

Why should the current division of roles be written in stone? All through history humanity has responded to two seemingly opposite pulls: the division of labour and the coordination of distinct tasks. Any productive organization knows how to effectively divide labour into distinct tasks and coordinate the work of individuals to complete these tasks. That takes careful thought, planning, and cooperation, lest functions fall between the cracks of job descriptions if there is a lack of clarity about when one professional's role stops and another one's starts.

Health care workers want to work at the top of their skills. Too often they are stymied by existing (and often ossified) rules and routines, especially in (but not only in) hospitals. Too often new roles are created to meet new needs instead of expanding existing roles, causing even more coordination problems. The kind of system design that leaves a gap between what a professional has the skill to do and what he or she is allowed to do produces waste. It also becomes a supply problem when high-level skills limited to existing roles are in short supply. Fortunately, expansion of existing roles is happening more frequently, a trend we heartily applaud.

Here is an example of role expansion. A Canadian woman vacationing in rural southern Italy experienced a bout of bladder infection. Having had a few of those, she knew she simply needed the right kind of antibiotics. In Canada that would have required a visit to the family doctor and probably a lab test, a prescription, and a visit to, or delivery from, a drug store for the physician-prescribed pharmaceutical. What should she do in rural Italy, where few people spoke English and where she wasn't familiar with the medical routines? Moreover, she fell ill on a Saturday. But the problem got solved in short order. The owner of her vacation home drove her to the nearest village (about 7,000 people), rang the doorbell of her own physician, who wasn't home, left a cellphone message on that doctor's phone, then drove the woman to a pharmacy and explained the problem to a pharmacist for her Canadian visitor. The pharmacist gave the Canadian woman two antibiotic powders, one to be taken right there and the other in 12 hours. Just then the physician returned the vacation homeowner's cellphone call. He listened to the story and told the landlady that the pharmacist would know what to do. The Canadian woman learned there and then that physicians were not the only ones who can prescribe drugs. The whole episode took less than an hour. Moreover, the two doses of the drug cured the infection within 24 hours. All the woman had to pay was about 11 euro ($14) for the pharmaceutical.

In Canada, that same woman has to make a doctor's appointment every three months to have her prescriptions renewed, a routine activity that takes her half a day (the time required to travel to her doctor's office, sit and wait for her appointment, talk to the doctor, and then travel home). Unless there is a change in her medical condition that would require a conversation with the physician, this is a waste of her time. With many doctors already having to see too many patients, it is a waste also of the physician's skill. Why not simply enable the pharmacy to fill prescriptions when refills are routine? (As we write this in February 2012, we are pleased to learn that Alberta has announced steps in that direction.) Why not get nurse practitioners to keep an eye on patients who are taking the prescribed drugs and have not had any complications since their last visit, preferably in a primary care setting?

Both the Kirby and Romanow reports identified the need for role redesign. We think the health system has no choice but to use available staff to their maximum potential to meet future health care needs. This will require a broad redesign of care models. We need to clarify who does what now, whether each task needs to be done at all, and who should do what in the future. This is the most critical task in planning for a healthy workforce sustainable for years to come.

Here are some of the things we see coming:

- Nurses will take on some roles that were previously the preserve of physicians.
- Health care aides or licensed practical nurses will take on roles previously reserved for registered nurses.
- Some jobs will expand beyond their current boundaries: nurse practitioners will have expanded roles in remote areas; pharmacists will provide prescriptions and administer immunizations, nurse practitioners will have an expanded role in critical care, and nurses will perform endoscopies.

Collaborative Practice

If Canadians' needs for chronic care and rehabilitation (the two main areas in which health care needs will increase in the near future) are to be met, new forms of working will be required. Many health care providers already possess some of the required skills in communication, assessment, care planning, implementation, and monitoring, although each profession may use a somewhat different vocabulary and framework. Each profession also has its own unique skill set. Nurses manage wounds and control infection, physiotherapists have expertise in mobility, occupational therapists help adapt environments, and social workers help to set up family support. However, they all need an appreciation for, and perhaps a minimal competency in, other disciplines, perhaps at some "assistant" level mentored by other professionals. When they work in interdisciplinary teams, professionals can improve their understanding of the skill sets of other team members, and communication problems when one discipline takes over a patient's care from another may be reduced. It also will reduce the number of visiting professionals and improve continuity of care and client satisfaction. In addition, it may address the supply problems in certain professions.

Role Substitution and Supplementation

A new interdisciplinary care model would involve changes in tasks or roles, as well as additions to existing ones. Pharmacists and nurses could assume some roles now reserved for physicians, for instance. However, while some authors have advanced proposals (even lists), and existing evaluations have documented the benefits of role or task substitutions to care, other studies have been more cautious about the impact on costs. Cost reductions cannot be the only reason for adopting a new interdisciplinary care model.

Given that nurses make up the largest component of the health care team in Canada (and in other countries), role changes will affect them most. Some progress has been made, but some barriers to effective changes still exist. For instance, there should be no barrier preventing nurse practitioners from discharging patients from hospitals and performing some other complex tasks.

Of course, some professional groups will react negatively to any role change proposals that would affect the existing hierarchies. All professions get involved in battles over turf. Fortunately, many individual health care professionals recognize that the existing structures are not capable of meeting Canadians' chronic care and rehabilitation requirements around the corner. There is too much unplanned and ad hoc role overlap now, especially with respect to nurses, leaving many health care workers feeling confused, undervalued, and not respected for their contributions. Many cross-sectional studies show that a richer nursing staff mix produces better health care outcomes. What is the ideal mix of registered nurses, practical nurses, and health care aides in hospitals? What should and can be done when there is a shortage of registered nurses? What is the impact of shifting some tasks to the two other types of professionals? What is the impact of decreasing the number of patients per nursing unit?

Importance of Productivity

Productivity has to do with the amount of time required to complete a given task. Productivity depends not only on the individual worker's skills but also on how their work is organized, the type of technology provided to them, and the input they receive from "upstream" and "downstream" professionals. Given current levels of productivity, Canada's aging and increasing population (Canada accepts roughly 250,000 new immigrants each year) will require substantial future increases in the number of health care workers. Statistics Canada predicts that Canada's population will steadily increase by around 10% every ten years. How many additional health care providers will be needed? Will we have enough of them? Studies show that even a small increase in productivity can have a major impact on the number of health care workers required.

Measuring productivity in health care is tricky. We're talking not simply about worker hours per patient. As we have pointed out several times already, health care outcomes are a vital component of any measurement in the health care system.

One other factor to be considered is the integration of new

recruits into a profession. New graduates may not be able to find even part-time work right away or may not be made to feel welcome when they find a job. They may become disillusioned and leave the profession after a short time. The nursing profession has a high rate of attrition in the early years of practice. Graduate programs and mentorship programs are excellent tools to halt or slow down attrition.

How Many Staff of Which Kind?

Workforce planning in health care depends on having a solid care model in place. Unfortunately, health care workplace planning has a poor track record, and physician needs planning is a good example. The current shortage of family physicians has its roots in the restrictions that were placed on the number of spots for students in medical faculties years ago. A mechanical approach (we have x family doctors now, and given increases in our population we will need y family doctors in the future) is inadequate. As we have pointed out before, care is changing, and the changes will require different mixes of health care providers. What is needed right now is careful consideration of future requirements, using alternate models incorporating alternate assumptions to be tested. Predictions of future requirements should also include assumptions about skill mixes, levels of productivity, and hours of work.

Who should lead this planning? We suggest that, given new health care models, planning should be led by those who have the responsibilities for health care delivery, rather than universities or colleges and professional associations.

We'd like to make one more point on staffing. Canada and its provinces have come to rely on internationally educated professionals. Imported nurses counted for 6.5% of the nursing workforce in 2005, and imported physicians for 22% of the total number of physicians. There are ethical concerns about such a dependency on foreign-trained workers; for instance, we may be luring health care providers from places that need them as well. Of course, a certain amount of international flow is natural: workers often migrate for family and personal reasons as well as for further training. However, a wealthy country such as Canada should aim to become self-sufficient, with in- and out-flows in balance. We therefore suggest that:

Provinces should model the workforce planning requirements for the larger health professions at least every five years. Health Canada should support the provinces by providing a national approach to model the workforce planning requirements for the smaller health professions. The larger provinces and the nation as a whole should aim for net self-sufficiency.

The Supply Side

The supply of health care professionals in Canada has been growing. Over the last ten years the number of nurses has increased by over 1% per year, and the number of physicians has increased at any even faster rate. The major strategies to increase supply have been to increase the number of students who enter university and college health care programs and the number of students who graduate from these programs. As we have argued, however, planning should be more comprehensive. It should begin with reflections on the skill sets that will be required in the future. It must then take into account role substitutions and extensions, the hours of care for which each type of professional is needed (e.g., physicians, registered nurses, practical nurses, and health care aides); in short, planners should look at joint requirements rather than the requirements for a single profession. Moreover, attention should be paid to the sources for increasing supply. For instance, there has been a steady trend over the past twenty years for physicians to restrict their hours of work. Incentives for part-time work should be considered, which would encourage more women with children to participate in the health care workforce and entice workers to stay in the workforce longer.

Expanding University and College Places

The traditional solution to workforce supply problems was to increase the number of places in universities and colleges, but this is not likely to work for the next decade. Population projections show a decline in the number of Canadians aged 15–19 and 20–24 years; these are the usual age groups of university and college entrants. That will put pressure on academic institutions to compete for candidates. A second problem concerns the difficulty of recruiting qualified faculty to staff the training programs for most health professions. There are strategies to address these problems, including academic innovation, greater cooperation between institutions to facilitate faculty development, and special funding.

Increasing Access to Health Care Professional Education

At the moment there is a disconnect between the profile of the people who enter professional health care education and the profile of the people they will come to serve. On the whole, entrants are richer, less ethnically diverse, and more likely to come from urban areas than the Canadian population in general. That is not an ideal situation, as physicians whose entire life experience has been in a city may not fully understand the issues faced by patients who live and work in rural communities. This rather narrow recruitment base may also come under pressure as the number of entrant positions in university and college programs is reduced.

Health professional education is not cheap. Many students and graduates face considerable debt on graduation. The spectre of higher debt loads will affect who applies to medical schools. Quebec has lower medical school fees than other provinces, and it also has more medical students from low-income neighbourhoods and whose parents have lower incomes. Other evidence concerning the link between the cost of professional education and the enrolment of students from low income groups is somewhat mixed. This suggests that a combination of strategies is needed to improve the diversity of student bodies. Contingent loans are one such strategy; these are loans linked to achievements. To increase staffing in rural and remote areas, contingent loans may be combined with debt forgiveness. These are good reasons to suggest that:

The federal government should explore with the provinces the possibility of developing a national income-contingent loan program for health professions, coupled with loan forgiveness to fill positions in hard-to-recruit areas.

Expanding Recruitment of Support Workers

The care model design we have advocated all through this book to respond to Canada's chronic care needs and our aging population will require an increasing number of health care aides and other support staff. Some studies suggest that we will need a steady increase of 1% or more annually for the foreseeable future. What strategies could be used to achieve this?

Many future health care roles will require less extensive training. Alberta initiated a certification program for health care aides who had received a minimum of three months' training. Their initial training allows health care aides to undertake a broader range of tasks, giving nurses and supervisors more room to delegate. Recognition (certification) of training also provides greater stability in the workforce, an important point where economies are volatile.

Alberta Health Services explored inviting older and middle-aged unemployed people to take this training as a way to enable them to enter or re-enter the workforce. With the costs of training recouped from employers, training became accessible to low-income people. Along with providing a new source of recruitment, this initiative had the added benefit of moving people from unemployment to employment.

A carefully planned and executed entry-level care program invites recruits to consider becoming a licensed practical nurse and possibly a registered nurse down the road. Distance education is becoming a powerful tool to provide in-home education and should be supported by employers as part of their regular staff development.

The Larger Context

In Canada health care is very public. Health care professionals are accountable in all directions, some formal and others informal, some explicit and others implicit. The less formal the accountability, the weaker it will be. The usual pressures come from six sides:

1   Health care professionals are accountable downward to the people they may employ. Employees hold their bosses accountable for providing reasonable working conditions and being fair in their expectations and performance assessments.

2   Health care professionals are also accountable upward (and sideways) to the people who employ them. When they are employees, they have to deal with management and hierarchies. As clinicians they are members of professional organizations that exert peer

pressure (sideways) through local hospital meetings and professional registration bodies. As the new health care design takes shape, accountability to multi-disciplinary colleagues will be an important factor.

3 To the "east" lurk provincial politicians, whose political demands may be unreasonable and whose propensity to take responsibility is highly suspect.

4 To the "south" the media are ready to pounce on any story that looks bad, even if it isn't.

5 To the "west," patient expectations are arrayed along many axes, from reasonable to unreasonable, from knowledgeable to ignorant.

6 To the "north," family and friends expect attention from people who work in physically and psychologically demanding jobs.

Implicit in this picture is our appreciation for the work of health care professionals. We have come to recognize that the stress of the system is directly related to the stress of their jobs, and we take our hats off to them.

Labour mobility bears upon the need for effective relationships between provincial registration boards. The efforts to make Canada an interprovincial free-trade country have moved slowly and ponderously and have been fraught with turf protection. The problems can be solved, and if the will exists this can be done easily. We recommend that:

Federal, provincial, and territorial leaders should review current health professional regulatory structures to facilitate further inter-provincial migration and provision of health care across provincial borders.

In conclusion, the sustainability of our medicare also depends on whether an appropriate workforce will be in place to meet future needs. It can be, provided that health systems and health education systems, as well as the health professions, are willing to make changes. It will take careful redesign work, and staff will need to be equipped with the skills they need for the new health care.

Tips for you:
- Does your province have a health workforce plan (either of its own or with neighbouring provinces)? What does it say about changes in roles?
- If you work in the health system, what sorts of role changes do you think are sensible for your work?

CHAPTER 11

Medicare Voices

Right from the first page we have maintained that Canada has a good medicare and that it can be sustained without crippling cutbacks or exorbitant taxes, but that it needs fine-tuning. Fine-tuning means making it more efficient, which entails both being cost conscious and providing (or enabling) the proper care.

Not all Canadians are convinced (yet) that medicare can be sustained even if we fine-tune it. Some are not convinced for ideological reasons: anarchists think that we should have no governments at all; libertarians want to dramatically shrink governments and government systems of care for those who need care. It is hard to dialogue with out-and-out ideologues, so we won't try. Others are (not yet?) convinced that the data provide a solid basis for optimism. In this chapter we let some of both the optimists and pessimists speak, and we'll respond to some of their concerns.

There is no shortage of proposals and think tank reports. Their conclusions depend on the lens used to view the system. They address these questions:

1 Is the Canadian health system in crisis?
2 If so, should it become more private?

It's useful to have a brief look at the past. Two major reviews of the health system were conducted in preparation for the 2004 accord: the Romanow report was a Royal Commission report and the Kirby report was a Senate report.

Kirby Report

The Kirby report was released in October 2002 after a two-year review by the Senate Standing Committee on Social Affairs, Science and Technology. Chaired by Liberal senator Michael Kirby, the report was supported by all committee members: seven Liberals, three Progressive Conservatives, and one independent.

The Kirby report presented a number of recommendations to promote efficiency, grounded in a move toward activity-based funding. It explicitly endorsed the concept of private provision of health care but embodied the belief that the "overwhelming majority" of institutional providers would remain either public or non-profit. It also strongly supported the maintaining of a single, public, funder of medicare. Here is what it said: "The Committee is keenly aware that shifting more of the cost to individual parents and their families via private payments, the facile 'solution' recommended by many, is really nothing more than an expensive way of relieving, or, at the least, diminishing governments' problem. Regardless of how it is expressed (as a share of gross domestic product (GDP), share of government spending, etc.) there is only one source of funding for health care – the Canadian public – and it has been shown conclusively that the most cost-effective way of funding health care is by using a single (in our case, publicly administered or governmental) insurer/payer model" (Kirby 2002, 9).

The report proposed expanding public responsibility and funding into new areas of health care, such as home care and pharmaceuticals. It also proposed a health care guarantee, recommending that "for each type of major procedure or treatment, a maximum needs-based waiting time be established and made public. When this maximum time is reached, the insurer (government) pays for the patient to seek the procedure or treatment immediately in another jurisdiction, including, if necessary, another country (e.g., the United States)."

Romanow Report

Released a few weeks after the Kirby report, the Romanow report was bolder and more expansionary. In Romanow's mandate the review context was clear: endorsement of the principles of the *Canada Health Act* and the strong attachment Canadians have to their medicare. The title of the report reflected that context: "Building on Values." For Romanow, health care was not just another commodity, but rather it was part of what it is to be a Canadian, a commitment Canadians make to each other, part of the glue that binds Canadians together in a compassionate society. With the 40th anniversary of medicare in mind, Romanow argued that "the next big step for Canada may be more focused, but it will be no less bold. That next step is to build on this proud legacy and transform medicare into a system that is more responsive, comprehensive and accountable to Canadians."

He issued this challenge: "Getting there requires leadership. It requires us to change our attitudes on how we govern ourselves as a nation. It requires an adequate, stable and predictable commitment to funding and co-operation from governments. It requires health practitioners to challenge the traditional way they have worked in the system. It requires all of us to realize that our health and wellness is not simply a responsibility of the state but something we must work for as individuals, families and communities, and as a nation. The national system I speak about is clearly within our grasp. Medicare is a worthy national achievement, a defining aspect of our citizenship and an expression of social cohesion. Let's unite to keep it so" (Romanow 2002, xxi).

The 2004 accord did respond to this challenge in part and delivered a "stable and predictable commitment to funding." But is funding ever totally adequate? In chapters 5 and 10 especially we have argued that the health professions have not yet sufficiently responded to the challenges directed their way.

Romanow's recommendations covered health care areas that are still weak:

- home care should be expanded;
- access should be improved; and
- electronic health records should be implemented.

Some of his recommendations were adopted (the Health Council of Canada and Canada Health Transfer were established); others have been adopted in modified form (waiting times initiatives). Some have yet to see any action (catastrophic drug provision, home care).

Romanow also addressed the contentious issue of the role of private enterprise. He distinguished between direct care, which he thought should be exclusively in the not-for-profit domain, and ancillary support services (e.g., food preparation, cleaning, and laundry), which he felt could be offered privately. He argued that the quality of ancillary support services could easily be measured and controlled and that these functions had no direct bearing on quality care. Whether his second claim is entirely valid is open to some debate.

Stakeholders

Since the release of the Kirby and Romanow reports and the signing of the 2004 accord, others have presented proposals. Among these are the views of stakeholders. Canada's health sector is the country's largest employer nationally, provincially, and often locally. For instance, Alberta Health Services is the 4th or 5th largest employer in all of Canada and the largest in the province; it employs people in practically every city and town of the province. Employee and professional groups have a critical stake in its future. Their voices are emerging as the expiry date of the 2004 accord approaches.

In 2010 the Canadian Medical Association published its prescription for health care transformation. It endorsed the five principles of the *Canada Health Act* and proposed two additions: patient-centredness and sustainability. Specifically, it proposed:

- a patient charter;
- changed incentives to enhance timely access and to support quality care;
- a new pharmaceutical scheme;
- enhanced access to continuing care;
- more effective workforce planning;
- more effective adoption of health information technologies; and
- better system accountability.

The Canadian Nurses Association established an expert commission to formulate its position. The Canadian Federation of Nurses Unions in its first contribution emphasized the important health system role of nurses and focused on nurse-specific issues. The Canadian Healthcare Association has also put forward its views.

Although there are differences in emphasis and language, key stakeholders seem to be united in their perception of the limitations of the current health care framework. They agree on many proposed directions for improvement. None of them calls for the extension of private funding. All four groups identify prevention, primary care, and home care as investment priorities.

Think Tanks and Policy Shops

A number of think tanks and policy shops have recently advanced their proposals for health system change. These tend to focus on financing issues rather than on service issues. Their vocabulary includes words like "crisis" and "unsustainability." It is not likely that the average Canadian will have a taste for their views.

The C.D. Howe Institute

In 2011 the C.D. Howe Institute issued a paper co-authored by former governor of the Bank of Canada David Dodge and Richard Dion with the title "Chronic Healthcare Spending Disease." They reached the following conclusion:

> Even if we in Canada are incredibly successful in improving the productivity, efficiency and effectiveness of the healthcare system – our optimistic case – we face difficult but necessary choices as to how we finance the rising cost of healthcare and manage the rising share of additional income devoted to it ... some combination of the following actions will be necessary to manage the "spending disease."
>
> 1 A sharp reduction in public services, other than healthcare, provided by governments, especially provincial governments;
> 2 Increase taxes to finance the public share of health-care spending;
> 3 Increased spending by individuals on healthcare services that are currently insured by provinces, through some form of co-payment or through delisting of services that are currently publicly financed;
> 4 A major degradation of publicly insured healthcare

standards – longer queues, services of poorer quality
– and the development of a privately funded system
to provide better-quality care for those willing to pay
for it. (Dodge and Dion 2011, 11)

The Fraser Institute

In a 2011 report, the Fraser Institute also questioned the sustainability of medicare. It focused on provincial budget proportions devoted to health care. It observed that provincial strategies have already curtailed spending as demonstrated by longer waiting times and limitations on public access to new pharmaceuticals. It concluded that the principles of the *Canada Health Act* constrain provincial responses to various issues and advanced the following proposal: "the Federal government should temporarily suspend enforcement of the *Canada Health Act* for a five-year trial period to allow the provinces to experiment with new ways of financing medical goods and services" (Skinner and Rovere, 2011, 3).

This would allow the following:

- reintroduction of user charges over and above current government payments to providers;
- introduction of private insurance for services currently covered by medicare; and
- expansion of the role of for-profit providers.

TD Economics

TD Economics' 2010 report on health care in Ontario also highlighted sustainability challenges, and it called health care "the Pac Man of provincial budgets." But it did not support an expanded role for private funding, noting that this would simply shift costs and wouldn't be politically achievable in any event. However, it advocated an expanded role for private sector provision. It is important to note that it offered a set of proposals for promoting more healthy lifestyles.

To improve efficiency, it proposed changing the way doctors are compensated, adopting activity-based funding, increasing bulk purchases of drugs, and imposing a health care benefit tax.

The Organisation for Economic Co-operation and Development

The Organisation for Economic Co-operation and Development (OECD) publishes a survey of member nations every other year. The most recent one about Canada was released in 2010. It reviewed Canada's economy and highlighted our health care. It lauded some aspects of it and called our medicare services top-notch, but it identified problems related to non-covered services, cost pressures, and waiting lists. On those it used strong language: "In the longer run the soundness of Canada's finances will likely largely be determined by the decisions taken regarding the health-care system ... With health already accounting for around half of total primary provincial spending, meeting the fiscal and demographic challenges will require that the growth of public health spending be reduced from an annual rate of about 8% seen over the last decade towards the trend rate of growth of nominal income in coming years (estimated to be less than 4% per year), the only alternative being to squeeze other public spending or to raise taxes or user charges" (Organisation for Economic Co-operation and Development 2010, 17).

Even so, the survey recommended expansion of the scope of services covered by the "core public package" (home care being the most notable addition), but it also recommended expansion of private funding through private insurance and co-payments.

In recent years the OECD has also published a series of comparative health system performance reports that use a statistical technique known as data envelopment analysis. It measures how far a country is away from a technically feasible frontier (the ideal within grasp, so to speak), identifying both output inefficiency (thereby indicating gains that could be made) and input inefficiency (indicating whether we can decrease input without losing desirable outputs). Canada has potential in both dimensions, as we have already argued in detail in our consideration of systems (primary care, home care, and hospitals).

The virtue of these OECD reports is that countries can learn from each other, for instance about life expectancy, one of the key output measures those reports use. Although Canada does relatively well, it lags behind the United States, the United Kingdom, Belgium, and the OECD average.

OECD researchers addressed the potential for efficiency improvement focusing on per capita health expenditures. All countries surveyed have seen these expenditures rise as a percentage of gross domestic product. Over the decade 1997–2007, Canada's per capita health expenditures increased 45%, just below the OECD average of 48%. Without the kind of changes we have outlined, Canada can expect a similar pattern for 2007–17.

The OECD also estimated the impact of changed policies and practice patterns. For example, Canada has longer average hospitalization stays for cancer than the OECD average. It suggested that with stronger primary care gatekeeping and less reliance on physician fee for service, Canada could achieve better value for money and meet projected demand with a smaller per capita increase in spending, perhaps as much as 5% less, and a resulting decrease in GDP spending of 2.5%.

Some Common Themes and Our Responses

First of all, we'll respond to some of the arguments that medicare is not sustainable. We specifically addressed this issue in chapters 2 and 3. Canada's population will age gradually, and we will have time to adapt to this demographic shift. Sustainability will also be affected by the introduction of enhanced health care (more technology, new services). Choices about introducing new technologies and services cannot, and should not, be made without considering funding options, which will include pursuits of greater social efficiencies and require political decision making about priorities.

A second theme in the arguments is pessimism about the potential to affect future expenditure needs with improved efficiency. We are optimistic about this, as we have demonstrated especially in chapters 4–10. For example, in the late 1990s Ontario established a Health Services Restructuring Commission, which, in spite of legal challenges and some adverse community reactions, produced positive changes. Here is what key participants observed: "Perhaps the most important [achievement] is that, for the time being at least, [the commission] broke the mold of the *status quo ante*. By exercising its power, [the commission] demonstrated that it is possible to make changes to health care – or at least restructure hospitals" (Sinclair et al. 2005, 213).

More recently, the creation of Alberta Health Services led to significant reductions in administrative layers and hundreds of millions of dollars in savings through centralization.

The third theme running through the proposals for change relates to the role of the private sector. Only the stakeholder reactions and the Romanow report did not recommend a greater role for private care providers, now or in the future. The Kirby report drew attention to what it described as the misunderstanding of the fifth principle of the *Canada Health Act*, namely public administration. The phrasing of the principle covers administration and is not about service delivery arrangements. Private delivery is already a major part of medicare, given that the vast majority of physicians are independent entrepreneurs. A range of medical services are also provided privately (e.g., cosmetic surgery, emergency medical services, pharmaceuticals, and dental care).

If we look at the issue of universal coverage, we see that public financing covers only the core medicare services: hospitals, physicians, and a range of diagnostic services. Some provinces provide additional publicly funded services for some groups (e.g., services for veterans and drug coverage for seniors). Hospital services are overwhelmingly publicly provided, although there are many not-for-profit hospitals owned by religious foundations, and some private services are supplied under contract to the public sector.

Emergency medical services (think ambulances) are primarily delivered by the public sector; sometimes they are funded by public sources but also through private insurance companies, and sometimes patients pay for them out of their own pockets. In a similar way, pharmaceuticals can also be funded publicly or privately. However, delivery of drugs is almost entirely private.

To repeat, private delivery is already a major part of medicare, although often in the public's mind public hospital care looms as the largest delivery system. Perhaps the apparent confusion could be resolved by updating the language of the *Canada Health Act* to focus on the word "governance," which carries a stronger meaning than the word "oversight." We therefore recommend that:

> The public administration criterion in the Canada Health Act *should be rephrased to reflect public governance and public financing.*

We sum up as follows:

- Romanow and stakeholders want to hold the line on private delivery as well as private financing.
- Kirby and TD Economics want to hold the line on private financing but expand private delivery.
- The C.D. Howe Institute and the Fraser Institute want to expand both private financing and delivery.

Private Financing

A number of arguments have been advanced for expanding private financing. Sometimes these arguments have inconsistencies. For instance, some propose increases in user charges, arguing that out-of-pocket payment is a strong incentive for patients to cut down on unnecessary use of health services. However, this argument is usually coupled with a call for more private insurance, which would dampen (or eliminate) any direct price signal effect on consumers.

There is a robust literature on user charges, which includes the RAND health insurance experiment in the United States. The report on this experiment concluded the following:

- user charges change utilization patterns;
- user charges have a greater impact on the poor than on the wealthy; and
- people whose behaviour changes as a result of user charges reduce both necessary and unnecessary care (the necessity of care is judged by professionals).

Those conclusions are to be expected. User charges are typically flat fees per visit. When you consider that people in lower income groups are often in poorer health than wealthier people and that user fees will eat up proportionally more of a poorer person's income, the conclusion is clear: it is an inequitable system.

Moreover, are there clear distinctions between necessary and unnecessary care? Consumers are not always good judges of what signs or symptoms indicate serious problems. User charges that discourage people from visiting a physician may lead to delays in essential care and hence to increased costs subsequently.

Universal health care ensures equity by having the healthy share costs with the sick and the rich share costs with the poor. User charges are in direct conflict with the principle of equity. Canadians know this, and hence politicians know this also. Consequently there is no broad support for the introduction of user fees. However, the temptation to go in this direction keeps popping up: "Like zombies in the night, these ideas may be intellectually dead but are never buried. They may be dormant for a time ... but when stresses build up either in the health care system or in the wider public economy, they rise up and stalk the land" (Evans et al. 1994, 1).

Insurance

An alternative to user charges is social insurance. With social insurance, health care is financed not with taxes but with a system of compulsory insurance with policies bought from for-profit insurance companies. That is the system in some countries, notably the Netherlands. High-income groups prefer voluntary insurance, but it establishes different access levels and may affect public provision of health care, which goes counter to the *Canada Health Act.*

Wider use of health insurance for services that are currently provided publicly is a prelude to the development of private markets in health care, guiding a greater proportion of the population to greater access to private services. But private markets for health care do not exist in Canada (or elsewhere), at least for necessary care. Evans tells us that "there is in health care no 'private, competitive market' of the form described in economic textbooks, anywhere in the world. There never has been, and the inherent characteristics of health and health care make it impossible that there ever could be" (Evans 1997, 428).

Why not? Social security insurance is such a complex business that it may well beyond the ability of most countries to enact the necessary regulatory framework. Risk management would be too complex, and the relevant technology is still a long way from being sufficiently developed. Recent social insurance reforms in the Netherlands were intended to strengthen competitive forces in social insurance, but there appears to have been little consumer response to the new "freedoms," partly because consumers did not, and perhaps could not, get the information they needed to confidently switch from one company to another.

The allure of social insurance is being kept alive, but Evans concludes that "[social insurance] costs more, yields no better average health outcomes, reduces participation in the formal labour force and, in developing countries, typically falls far short of universality" (Evans 2009, 23). Other observers agree.

Private versus Public Spending

The advocates for increased private spending often claim that this will take the pressure off public spending. But are public and private spending substitutes for each other? The facts suggest that this is not the case.

A 2008 OECD study on health care spending of selected countries found that Canada's private spending on health care accounted for roughly 3% of its GDP and public spending for just over 7% of its GDP. The United States, where private spending accounted for close to 9% of GDP, still devoted roughly 7.5%

of its GDP to public spending, a higher percentage than Canada. In Norway, the country with the highest per capita GDP, just over 7% of its GDP was used for public spending, but private spending accounted for just over 1%.

As GDP increases over time, so does health care spending, driven primarily by an increase in public spending. The United States is an anomaly among the nations in the report. For all others public spending was strongly correlated with per capita GDP, and the correlation between private spending and GDP was weak. However, for both the United States and Norway the correlation was almost non-existent.

Although for all other countries (with the exception of Norway), there seemed to be a predictable relationship between GDP increases and public health care outlay, the United States' experience is a lesson for us all. Its public spending as a percentage of GDP is close to expectations given the size of its GDP, but its far greater total spending as a percentage of GDP is driven entirely by its excess private spending. In short, there is no evidence to suggest that private spending takes the place of public spending. Increasing the portion of private spending is a risky proposition indeed. In Canada it may not deliver the promised financial benefits, and it will certainly undermine equity. As one wit suggested, the greatest threat to Canada's medicare may be this attempt to save it. Expanding private share is almost certainly a damaging move. Therefore,

> *Canadian health care is best served by a continuation of tax financing, and expansion of private insurance into core areas should not be pursued.*

Private versus Public Delivery

Private funding of health care is a fairly small portion of total health care funding in Canada; private delivery of health care is a much more significant portion of total delivery. Private companies supply laboratory medicine and diagnostic imaging, most physicians run private practices for which they bill provincial governments, and a goodly proportion of long-term care is provided by for-profit companies. There is no strong sentiment for changing the use of for-profit laboratories and imaging companies, although contracts are always subject to negotiations to ensure that benefits from greater efficiencies also accrue to the public and that these services offer sufficient quality. (By contrast, for-profit surgical facilities seem more contentious.)

Private delivery and private financing are two separate, and not necessarily linked, concepts. We can maintain public financing and have private delivery. A number of arguments have been advanced for increasing private delivery. For instance, private delivery will facilitate innovation and produce greater efficiency. That may be true for many businesses that operate in a free market with the following givens:

- the market is not monopolistic; and
- the businesses' internal workings must not be dependent on a massive flow of information, to prevent costly mistakes including the loss of life.

These assumptions do not hold in health care. For instance, hospitals have a local monopoly and their information costs are very high. Arguments for private delivery are clearly ideological and not based on reality. The results of detailed studies comparing the benefits of private and public hospitals in both the United States and Germany are a mixed bag: some suggest that a private (for profit) model is preferable and others indicate that a public model is preferable. In one study, mortality outcomes were worse in for-profit facilities than in not-for-profit ones.

Contracting

For private delivery within a public framework, well-specified contracts must be in place that state precisely which services are to be delivered. Setting up such contracts is anything but a trivial task, and fortunately the last decade has seen an improvement in how hospitals can be described in terms of the patients they treat. On the other hand, it remains difficult to also describe standards of quality. Recent work by some economists has focused on the problems of deciding whether to buy products or services or produce them. What is involved when there is only one company producing a vital product (a monopoly)? How do you have a competitive market when the provision of the service requires a big building that cannot be used for anything else, a condition called asset specificity? The latter undermines the rhetoric of the market economy and its assumption that there will be many competing products and companies. This situation also opens the door to political interference.

Poorly designed contracts may lead to public purchasers overpaying private providers. Moreover, gains in efficiency may accrue to the providers only. Good contracts are not yet the norm in all of Canada.

Private delivery of health care has the potential to produce benefits in Canada, notably in the stimulation of innovation and improved efficiency. On the other hand, it carries risks of overpayment and an unhealthy dependency on asset-specific suppliers.

This entire book is grounded in the premise that the Canadian health care system needs to change. One problem concerns the very use of the term "Canadian health care system." There isn't one. There are many: one in each province and territory. Even more problematic is the fact that "no province, nor Canada as a whole, has a [health care system], if we take the word system to mean an organization in which the many different and diverse parts function together" (Sinclair et al. 2005, 23).

Our conclusions are as follows. Canada does not yet have a high-performing health care system. It may well be better than many alternatives. Access is better than in the United States and our health care system overall is far superior. In both countries you can find pockets of excellence, but we do not yet have a system in which *the right person enables the right care in the right setting, on time, every time.*

In our last chapter we describe how we might get there.

CHAPTER 12

The Road Ahead

In chapters 2 and 3 we argued that Canadian medicare is sustainable. We looked at what's been happening and what needs to happen. The moment has come to point the way to a secure future for medicare. Of course we cannot guarantee that our "prescription" will be implemented or even that it will be followed. All we can do is put up signposts to point politicians, health care providers, and managers in the right direction. They are the ones who will make the required changes. Our hope is that this book will help many more Canadians to prod them effectively. All direct health care providers need to be pushed and held to account by media watchdogs and an alert public. We hope that this book will be a pushing instrument in the hands of Canadians who care for our medicare and want to see it flourish to the benefit of us all.

You may already have noticed the major themes running through the preceding chapters:

- We are concerned for disadvantaged populations.
- We have addressed needs as yet unmet.
- We prefer the least restrictive alternatives.
- We have consistently weighed three value perspectives: patient, clinician, and economy.
- We like using economic incentives.
- We recognize the potential of multiple provider forms.

Using existing resources to their maximum is the key. Our efficiency agenda is not simply about cutting costs or spending less. It is about using limited resources wisely:

- Every needed service is to be provided in the most efficient way.
- Every service provided responds to a genuine need.
- Every investment should improve outcomes.

This book contains many proposals for change, which we have compiled in appendix 1. Some are big, like coverage of pharmaceuticals, but most are small and incremental. The focus on incremental changes is no accident. First, our fundamentals are already in place. We don't need big bang reforms. Second, looking at implementation, the proposed changes are achievable. However, although many of the changes are small, it doesn't mean that the overall effect won't be profound. In fact, the effect will be so profound that we have no doubt that our medicare will continue to be sustainable.

The Levers of Change

Three levers control the engine of health care:

- financial levers and incentives;
- laws, regulations, and governance arrangements; and
- norms, culture, and people working together.

The evolution of the Canadian health care system, and the way it has responded to challenges, shows the strength of our people working together. This strength is a key to success, together with a mix of other instruments including top down performance instruments, mainly incentives and ways of governance, target setting, and performance assessments. We have also talked about challenges from below, which include user choices and activity-based funding.

Governance is important. Romanow observed ahead of the 2004 accord that stable and secure funding is an essential prerequisite for any change. The 2004 accord gave health care in Canada stability. Provinces knew in advance what funds would flow from the federal government and the criteria that would be used to judge the legitimacy of their actions.

The federal government announced in late 2011 that after an interim period of 6% increases, funding increases to the provinces in the future will be in line with growth in the economy. At first blush it may seem reasonable to restrict funding to what the economy can afford. However, the trend has been for health costs to grow faster than the growth rate of the economy, and in addition the government's new approach does not provide the certainty that the fixed 6% gave. The federal government is effectively transferring risk from Canadian federal taxpayers to provincial taxpayers (the same people, wearing different taxpayer hats).

In a tighter fiscal environment, some provinces may want to challenge some of the basic tenets of medicare. There needs to be continued reinforcement of the broad parameters within which provinces can manage medicare. The existing principles provide a well-accepted framework, but they may need to be revised slightly if the scope of medicare is expanded (e.g., to encompass home care and pharmaceuticals). In addition, the criterion of comprehensiveness should be clarified to address effectiveness and the public administration criterion should also be clarified (see chapters 7 and 9). Hence,

All federal and provincial proposals on health care should reaffirm the principles of the Canada Health Act *in a modified form.*

In previous chapters we have argued for changes in the federal role, and some of these will require increases in federal spending. Many proposals are inexpensive and can be routinely incorporated into future budgets. The exception is the pharmaceutical program, which will save costs in the end but will involve a redistribution of who spends what. Chapter 6 does not provide a definite proposal but gives the outlines of a process to create one, which would require a realignment of funding responsibilities between the federal and provincial governments.

Accountability and Transparency

Both the delivery and policy arms of the health care system should embrace the concept of continuous improvement. This requires a change from the current ways of doing things. First, there has to be a renewed emphasis on transparency regarding the performance of health care, both nationally and provincially. At present different provinces use different definitions for key performance indicators and they may withhold information that would be useful for national data banks. Although some progress has been made, key questions regarding health care performance in Canada cannot be answered until data gaps are filled in. In this respect Australia, which also has a federal system, does a much better job. Canada's data gaps mask transparency, inhibit accountability, and slow the process of educating one another across the country. As potential patients and active taxpayers we are not served as well as we could be.

Both accountability and transparency depend on common data definitions so that performance measures can be calculated across a range of dimensions, notably outputs (volume), outcomes (quality), and processes (access). Performance measures should be broad in scope, should recognize the multidimensional nature of health and health care objectives, and should address Canadians' concerns about performance (e.g., waiting times). The measures should have an evidence base and have credible benchmarks. Performance measures should be relevant to existing data collections, but they should also take into account the cost of new data collections. A road map will need to be developed to phase in new performance measures prompted by new data, for instance patient-reported outcome measures, as patient satisfaction is a component of productivity.

Linked Data Sets and Their Impact

We have already stressed the need for all provinces to learn from each other, as all of them must take the road toward greater economic and social efficiency. Linked data sets are a tool that can be used for this learning. Data collection is well underway in hospitals and other facilities, and the resulting data sets are being linked to each other. Some provinces already link various types of collected data to shine light on whole system performance. The Manitoba Centre for Health Policy is a leader in this regard, and its efforts are providing insight into system performance and efficiency directions. Ontario's Institute for Clinical Evaluative Sciences has also developed a successful model. But not all provinces have moved this far. For one thing, privacy concerns associated with linking data sets need to be addressed. However, for developing greater health care efficiency, the power of information must be harnessed for the benefit of us all. Linked data sets are an essential component of system learning. Information gathered in one place should be available to all, and across Canada.

Collecting data is one thing, acting on them is another. Early in this book we suggested that Canada's medicare is sustainable in the long run, but only if we begin to make changes now. Health care professionals, especially policy-makers, must find ways to use the information collected to get innovations and quality improvements underway without delay. The data arising from individual clinical experiences must not get lost in bureaucracies and information traffic jams. The roots of health care progress are data gathered in one place, but the roots must produce branches, flowers, and fruit. What will be needed is a "rapid learning health system," a way of getting knowledge into practice without delay. The work of the Manitoba Centre for Health Policy has demonstrated how the proper use of data can guide policy and practice at the provincial level, creating a new model for clinical effectiveness research.

Key to this rapid learning health system is the analysis of actual experiences with newly implemented treatments to assess outcomes and costs in real practice situations. This approach goes beyond the controlled environments and carefully selected patient populations that are characteristic of randomized controlled trials (the traditional, and slow, way to evaluate innovation). The approach depends on assessing patient outcomes at local levels and comparing those with average outcomes in other places within or beyond the province.

System Evaluation

We repeat: transparency and accountability should apply to all levels of the system. Policy-makers should no longer drop their decisions on operational folk; all policies should be up for review, evaluation, and critique. The 2004 accord was preceded by the 2002 Kirby and Romanow reports. Where is the interim review of that accord, which would serve as a platform for future official federal-provincial health care relationships and agreements? Given the many suggestions for innovations and improvements, it would be wise to aim for periodic comprehensive reviews prepared for, but independent of, federal and provincial governments.

The Need for Leadership and Innovation

A host of changes are needed to respond better to emerging health care needs and keep Canadian medicare sustainable. New ideas need to be embraced. In some sectors they already have been. Unfortunately, these ideas seem to be limited to clinical practices. As of yet there is no systematic approach to administrative, policy, and service innovation throughout Canada's health system.

Given the pressure on resources, it may be difficult to create room for long-term planning and research into new evidence-based management approaches. Moreover, to date, what may be useful evidence has been gathered not so much from the public sector as from the private sector. Context is important, so perhaps there is a serious knowledge gap for public service organizational learning. Finally, in many places clinical and administrative authorities may work in parallel but fairly unconnected ways, which may create difficulties with implementing changes. In a decentralized system such as ours, multiple players feel they can exercise veto power.

Traditionally, businesses live and die by innovation, but public sectors do not. The public sector tends to have lower turnover of personnel and it tends to work with poor measurements of quality and payment policies (linked most often not to value but to volume). Hence,

Provinces should build on the nationally agreed performance measures to develop clear performance measure for health and health care in the province and for every separately incorporated health delivery agency in the province.

and

Provinces should develop strategies for public reporting
of the performance of delivery agencies and processes to
build accountability for delivery agencies.

The Crucial Role of Provincial Leadership

In Canada provinces are responsible for providing health care, and much of the burden of health care reform falls therefore on provincial shoulders. Then again, the provinces will be the major beneficiaries of the positive results of improved efficiency. It should surprise no one that about half of our recommendations are directed at the provinces (see appendix 1). It may look like we are placing a lot of the responsibility for change with the provinces, but most of the suggestions will involve incremental change.

Reform has a mixed track record. Recognizing this, the OECD has established a Making Reform Happen project and has identified four factors that will either help or hinder reform:

- the availability of information, evidence, and analysis;
- the use of incentives (and disincentives);
- political leadership and political possibilities; and
- the availability of resources.

The first two have been richly described in this book. The third one is no secret. The fourth one may be addressed through political will. Political leadership and commitment are critical, can be influenced by stakeholders, can be supported by managers, and can be pushed by the public at large. Data can be assembled and techniques for analyzing and using data to effect change can be developed, but in the end politicians must be persuaded to act on the data and not on power and popularity impulses.

Public Participation and Involvement

Earlier we cited the work of others in suggesting that one of the major factors driving public sector reform is the influence of users shaping services from below. Patients' rights have become a talking point in Canada. The Canadian Medical Association recently proposed a Charter of Patients' Rights as a component of its reform proposals, and a Minister's Advisory Committee in Alberta has made a similar recommendation. Many health delivery agencies have developed formal mechanisms for user or public involvement. There is considerable debate about such involvement, and the following sorts of questions are being discussed:

1   *Why* should the public participate in health policy?
2   *Who* constitutes the public?
3   *What* health policy issues should be canvassed in exercises of public participation?
4   *Which* public participation methods are productive?

For a start,

Delivery agencies should review their current approaches to public participation to assess whether they are addressing contemporary needs. Provinces should establish guidelines for minimum standards of public participation. Health Canada should convene a conference every three years to share delivery agencies' experiences with public participation.

Conclusion

This book has told the essential story of medicare, describing its past, present, and future. With respect to past and present, the overall policy and character of medicare is sound. The institutional framework is appropriate. With respect to the future, medicare is sustainable.

But change is necessary. Our population and health have changed over the more than 50 years of medicare's existence. Our population is growing, on the whole we are aging, and health problems have changed. We must respond to new demands. However, in spite of the many complexities touched on in this book, we are not calling for a drastic overhaul but rather for incremental changes by every part of the system: clinicians, politicians, institutions, administrators, and also us, the users and patients. These changes are built on the strengths of what already exists, including the commitments and skills of providers and the commitments of Canadians to their medicare.

We're calling for greater efficiency, both in terms of economic and social efficiency. We must strengthen equality of access. We must improve the overall health of Canadians and extend life expectancy. It won't be easy. Change is uncomfortable. Some segments of our society will want to protect the status quo because it favours them.

But we are convinced that the vast majority of Canadians want a system that works, for us all and for us individually. The aim of this book has been to show one path for how that aspiration can become a reality.

A tip for you:
What opportunities are there for the public to shape health services in your province? Consider not just board positions (which are often reserved for the politically connected and are few and far between) but also local advisory committees. Apply to participate and take up the cudgels for a better system for yourself, your kids, and your neighbours.

Recommendations

This appendix lists all of the recommendations made in the chapters of this book.

From chapter 4:

- A pan-Canadian set of goals and targets for improving the health status of all Canadians should be developed by governments. Each province should publish its own goals and targets, consistent with the national goals and targets. Regional health authorities and other organizations should also consider the development of goals and targets consistent with the national goals and targets.
- Provinces and regional health authorities should publish regular reports on disparities in health outcomes.
- The Canadian Health Services Research Foundation should be given the task to review the evidence on the use of tax incentives to promote public health objectives, including the case for a targeted tax on sugar-sweetened beverages.

From chapter 5:

- The federal government should make available a personal health record platform for all Canadians; all provinces should work with Health Canada to

facilitate populating the personal health record with
provincially held data.

- Provinces should consider integration of home care
  and other community services with new (transformed) multidisciplinary primary care practices.
- Provinces should review payment arrangements for
  family physicians to ensure that these incorporate the
  right set of incentives for care of patients with chronic
  illnesses including incentives that encourage physicians to support self-management, community-level
  interventions, and the optimal division of labour.
- Provinces should review their primary care funding
  arrangements to ensure that funding streams are
  adequate to allow collaborative team practice.

From chapter 6:

- Prescription drugs should be an insured service under
  medicare. Federal, provincial, and territorial leaders
  should immediately commission an independent
  study of the most practicable way of introducing
  prescription pharmaceuticals as an insured service
  under medicare.

From chapter 7:

- Academic Health Science Centres should document
  and publicize to their students how their research
  actually leads to improvements in efficiency in the
  delivery of care.

From chapter 8:

- Provinces should incorporate self-managed care
  as an integral part of their home care systems.
- Seniors' health care, whether provided in the home
  or in a residential aged-care facility, should become

an insured service under the *Canada Health Act*.
- Provinces should explore the possibility of publicly reporting the quality of nursing home care.
- Provinces should encourage and facilitate development of a broader range of accommodation options for seniors, including an intermediate residential care option, assisted living.
- Provinces should aim for activity-based funding for residential care.

From chapter 9:
- The Canadian Patient Safety Institute should develop guidelines for incident reporting systems and mechanisms to share lessons from incident reviews across Canada.
- The Canadian Institute for Health Information should be given the task and be funded to expand publication of data on variation in utilization rates across Canada.
- Provinces should create and fund clinical networks to provide leadership in sharing good practice to improve access to health care and the quality and sustainability of health care.
- The comprehensiveness criterion in the *Canada Health Act* should be amended to include an obligation on the part of provinces to cover effective services, with a requirement that effectiveness be determined in a transparent way.
- Provinces should request clinical networks (when established) to review intra- and inter-provincial utilization rate differences. Networks should be invited to develop or update priority-setting criteria.
- Provinces should commit to adopting common definitions of waiting times for the full patient journey.

- Federal, provincial, and territorial leaders should agree to waiting time ranges for a broad range of services. Provinces should publish consistent data on their achievement of those targets at least quarterly; these data should be collated and published nationally by the Canadian Institute for Health Information at least annually.
- Provinces should commit to a phased introduction of activity-based funding to drive improvements in efficiency in the hospital sector and other sectors.

From chapter 10:
- Provinces should model the workforce planning requirements for the larger health professions at least every five years. Health Canada should support the provinces by providing a national approach to model the workforce planning requirements for the smaller health professions. The larger provinces and the nation as a whole should aim for net self-sufficiency.
- The federal government should explore with the provinces the possibility of developing a national income-contingent loan program for health professions, coupled with loan forgiveness to fill positions in hard-to-recruit areas.
- Federal, provincial, and territorial leaders should review current health professional regulatory structures to facilitate further inter-provincial migration and provision of health care across provincial borders.

From chapter 11:
- The public administration criterion in the *Canada Health Act* should be rephrased to reflect public governance and public financing.

- Canadian health care is best served by a continuation of tax financing, and expansion of private insurance into core areas should not be pursued.

From chapter 12:

- All federal and provincial proposals on health care should reaffirm the principles of the *Canada Health Act* in a modified form.
- Provinces should build on the nationally agreed performance measures to develop clear performance measure for health and health care in the province and for every separately incorporated health delivery agency in the province.
- Provinces should develop strategies for public reporting of the performance of delivery agencies and processes to build accountability for delivery agencies.
- Delivery agencies should review their current approaches to public participation to assess whether they are addressing contemporary needs. Provinces should establish guidelines for minimum standards of public participation. Health Canada should convene a conference every three years to share delivery agencies' experiences with public participation.

Key Canadian Health Organizations

• Canadian Federation of Nurses Unions (CFNU)
www.nursesunions.ca

The Canadian Federation of Nurses Unions is the national industrial (union) voice of registered nurses in Canada. It is a federation of provincial and territorial nursing unions.

• Canadian Health Services Research Foundation (CHSRF)
www.chsrf.ca

The Canadian Health Services Research Foundation brings researchers and decision makers together to create and apply knowledge to improve health services for Canadians. CHSRF is an independent, not-for-profit corporation, established with endowed funds from the federal government and its agencies and incorporated under the *Canada Corporations Act*. It produces good quality summaries of critical issues for Canadian health care, informed by research.

• Canadian Institute for Health Information (CIHI)
www.cihi.ca

The Canadian Institute for Health Information was established in 1994 as an independent, not-for-profit corporation
that provides information on Canada's health system and
the health of Canadians. You'll find lots of statistics on its
website.

• Canadian Medical Association (CMA)
www.cma.ca

The Canadian Medical Association is the national voice of
the medical profession. It is a federation of provincial and
territorial medical associations.

• Canadian Nurses Association (CNA)
www.cna-aiic.ca/cna

The Canadian Nurses Association is the national professional
voice of registered nurses in Canada. It is a federation of
provincial and territorial nursing associations and colleges.

• Canadian Public Health Association (CPHA)
www.cpha.ca

The Canadian Public Health Association is a national, independent, not-for-profit, voluntary association representing
the public health field in Canada.

• Health Canada
www.hc-sc.gc.ca

Health Canada is the federal department responsible
for health.

• Public Health Agency of Canada
www.phac-aspc.gc.ca/index-eng.php

The Public Health Agency of Canada is the main government
agency responsible for public health in Canada.

• Royal College of Physicians and Surgeons of Canada
www.royalcollege.ca

The Royal College of Physicians and Surgeons of Canada is
the national professional association that oversees the medical education of specialists in Canada. It accredits the university programs that train resident physicians for their specialty
practices and sets the examinations that residents must pass
to become certified as specialists.

Bibliography

Barer, M.L., R.G. Evans, and C. Hertzman. 1995.
"Avalanche or glacier?: Health care and the demographic
rhetoric." *Canadian Journal on Aging* 14(2):193–224.

Decter, M. 2007. "Chronic disease: Our growing challenge."
In J. Dorland and M.A. McColl, eds., *Emerging approaches
to chronic disease management in primary health care.*
Montreal and Kingston: Queen's Policy Studies and McGill-
Queen's University Press.

Dodge, D.A., and R. Dion. 2011. *Chronic healthcare spending disease: A macro diagnosis and prognosis.* Toronto:
C.D. Howe Institute.

Duckett, S. 2012. *Where to from here? Keeping medicare
sustainable.* Montreal and Kingston: Queen's Policy Studies
and McGill-Queen's University Press.

Evans, R.G. 1997. "Going for the gold: The redistributive
agenda behind market-based health care reform." *Journal
of Health Politics, Policy and Law* 22(2):427–65.

– 2009. "The iron chancellor and the fabian." *Healthcare
Policy* 5(1):16–24.

Forget, G., S.J. Taylor, S. Eldridge, J. Ramsay, and C.J. Grif-
fiths. 2007. "Self-management education programmes by
lay leaders for people with chronic conditions." *Cochrane
Database of Systematic Reviews* 4. CD005108.

Gagnon, M.-A. 2010. *The economic case for universal pharmacare: Costs and benefits of publicly funded drug coverage for all Canadians.* Ottawa and Montreal: Canadian Centre for Policy Alternatives and Institut de recherche et d'informations socio-économiques.

Kirby, M.J.L. 2001. *The health of Canadians – the federal role. Report of the Standing Senate Committee on Social Affairs, Science and Technology.* Ottawa: Senate of Canada.

Landon, S., M.L. McMillan, V. Muralidharan, and M. Parsons. 2006. "Does health-care spending crowd out other provincial government expenditures?" *Canadian Public Policy* 32(2):121–41.

Organisation for Economic Co-operation and Development. 2010. Canada. OECD *Economic Surveys* 2010(14).

Romanow, R.J. 2002. *Building on values: The future of health care in Canada – final report.* Ottawa: Commission on the Future of Health Care in Canada.

Sinclair, D.G., M. Rochon, and P. Leatt. 2005. *Riding the third rail: The story of Ontario's Health Services Restructuring Commission, 1996–2000.* Montreal: Institute for Research on Public Policy.

Stacey, D., C.L. Bennett, M.J. Barry, N.F. Col, K.B. Eden, M. Holmes-Rovner, H. Llewellyn-Thomas, et al. 2011. "Decision aids for people facing health treatment or screening decisions." *Cochrane Database Systematic Reviews.* Issue 10. Article CD001431. DOI: 10.1002/14651858.

Starfield, B. 1992. *Primary care: Concept, evaluation and policy.* New York: Oxford University Press.

Wagner, E.H., R.E. Glasgow, C. Davis, A.E. Bonomi, L. Provost, D. McCulloch, P. Carver, et al. 2001. "Quality improvement in chronic illness care: A collaborative approach." *Joint Commission Journal on Quality Improvement* 27(2):63–80.

Index